PRAISE FOR "STROKE! A DAUGHTER'S STORY"

— *"This book is beneficial to both patients and families to help them understand they are not alone, and that it's all right to have feelings of anguish, depression, anger and guilt. I believe every doctor should read this. I am quoting it to my nurses and want them to share it with patients, health care professionals and volunteers who deal with the family under trauma.*

Carol Pendleton, RN Nursing Coordinator, Oncology Dept., HCA Lawnwood Regional Medical Center, Ft. Pierce, FL Chairman of the Board, Hospice of Treasure Coast

— *"A monumental task clearly defining the physical and emotional turmoil caused by a CVA. Her book should bring comfort and reassurance to other families going through the stroke experience, and a greater understanding to physicians and therapists who have not had to confront the terror of this disease."*

Ross Dodge, Psychiatric Social Worker Visiting Nurse Association, Martin County, Stuart, FL

— *"Touching ... descriptive, and practical. A book to be read and reread for its helpful information about the stroke crisis. Truly a caregiver's handbook!"*

Gladys McCathern, Administrator Bortz Nursing Home, Hobe Sound, Florida

— *"This is a cry for help from the inexperienced caregiver who must take on the role of nurse, therapist, and guardian for the homebound stroke patient. Miss Thurston's book helps to fill the gap between the medical profession, our health care system and the stroke family, pointing out the need for 1) family education, 2) community involvement, and 3) Stroke Club Support Groups."*

Mary Chicca, President, Port St. Lucie Stroke Club, FL.

— *"Families of stroke victims can profit from each other's experience. This is one of few such books available written by the caregiver and should prove a valuable contribution to the medical field as well."*
  Martha Taylor Sarno, Speech Pathologist (aphasia)
  New York University Rehabilitation Medical Center
  Author: Stroke: The Condition and the Patient

— *"Perhaps this book will throw some light on the need — and ask the question, 'How can we help those who are victims of the victim? How can we, as individual and community, better care for our impaired elderly?"*
  Maggie Hurchalla, Martin County Commissioner (ret.)
  (Sister of the former Attorney General), Stuart, FL

— *"A moving, factual report, written from the heart, and communicating the despair and helplessness of family members in the stroke crisis. The book depicts the frustration, anguish, and very personal hell of a daughter in dealing with the "child-parent,' 'child-adult,' 'adult-adult' relationships and their most complex scripts. Doris Thurston bares her soul and shares in eloquent style, reaching out to ANY audience, especially health care professionals and caregivers who can gain empathy and insight."*
  Dr. Jean Sloan, DPA
  Director of Educational Services
  Martin Memorial Medical Center, Stuart, FL

— *"Your book is fascinating! I could not put it down. The drawings and poems are most effective. Your soul-searching torment adds an essential dimension. I can see the book being of greatest value to health care workers and families of stroke victims."*
  Mary Lou Hughes, ACSW
  Licensed Clinical Social Worker
  St. Lucie Home Health, Port St. Lucie, FL

— *"Enlightening. I don't feel so alone. . .You opened a window to my emotions and I now realize others go through the same negative emotions, so I don't have to feel so guilty! The death experience was beautifully portrayed and your reliance on spiritual values. I wanted it to continue. . ."*

Viola Koran, (Caregiver)
Treasure Coast Stroke Club
Stuart, FL

— *"Your book is spiritual! I find the poems challenging, provocative and inspirational. We can use them in our Stroke Club discussions."*

Adele Kates, Speech Pathologist,
Chair of the AHA Stroke Council,
and former director of the
Florida Stroke Convention, 1981

STROKE!
A Daughter's
Story

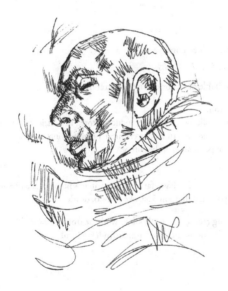

With Drawings
by the Author

DORIS THURSTON

Order this book online at www.trafford.com
or email orders@trafford.com

Most Trafford titles are also available at major online book retailers.

Stroke: A Daughter's Story
Summary: A daughter cares for her stroke-aphasic father in her parent's home over a five year period.
1. stroke 2. aphasia 3. caregiving 4. rehabilitation 5. stroke clubs 6. death

Note for Librarians: A cataloguing record for this book is available from Library
and Archives Canada at www.collectionscanada.ca/amicus/index-e.html

Printed in Victoria, BC, Canada.

ISBN: 978-1-4120-7875-7

*Our mission is to efficiently provide the world's finest, most comprehensive book publishing
service, enabling every author to experience success. To find out how to publish your book, your
way, and have it available worldwide, visit us online at www.trafford.com*

Trafford rev. 9/30/2009

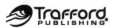 www.trafford.com

North America & international
toll-free: 1 888 232 4444 (USA & Canada)
phone: 250 383 6864 ♦ fax: 812 355 4082

OTHER BOOKS BY AUTHOR/ARTIST, DORIS THURSTON
(*Illustrated)

POETRY (Spiral Bound)
*Ausable Chasm
*Poem to Thoreau
*The Temple Within: Sonnets and Asanas
*Trauma to Triumph: Poems of a Caregiver
*Oh America! Memorial Poems to John F. Kennedy
* Song in the Woods
*The Beatitudes: Meditations and Prayers
Notes on Oskar Kokoschka
(as he taught at Boston Museum School of Art, 1949)

NON-FICTION (Perfect bound)
A WAC Looks Back: Recollections and Poems of WWII

*Available at The Women's Memorial, Washington, DC
(1-800-222-2294), and on-line at Amazon.com, Borders,
and Barnes and Noble*

FORTHCOMING: NON-FICTION
*A Yoga Tour of India with Swami Vishnu DeVenanda

*Available from Thurston Arts
842 SE St. Lucie Boulevard, Stuart, FL. 34996
(Tel) 772-283-5137, E-mail: dtStrokeBook@aol.com*

TO ROBERT RAY THURSTON,

My Father, who,
as a stroke-aphasic patient, taught us to love again.

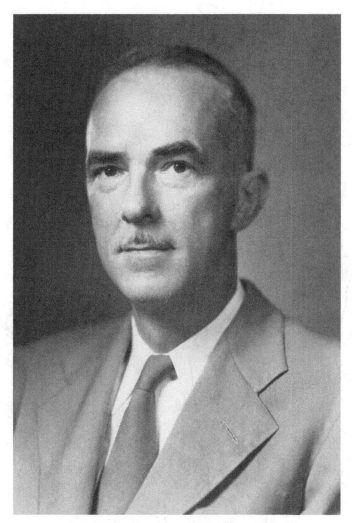

"But he knoweth the way that I take:
when he hath tried me, I shall come forth as gold."

Job 23:10

The Garden of Eden...

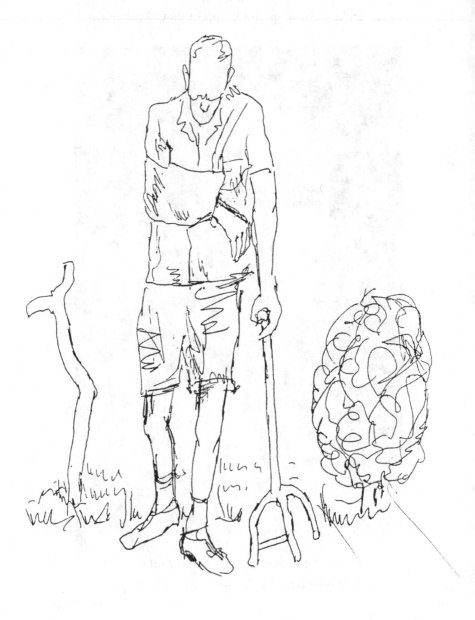

SUFFERING

Suffering turns the mind towards God.

Suffering infuses mercy in the heart

and softens it.

Suffering strengthens. . .

In the same way you get the scent

only by squeezing the leaves of

a walnut or verbena tree, you get

the essence out of people only

when

they are suffering—or in trouble.

Therefore Suffering is a blessing

in disguise.

It is the only best thing in

this world.

Master Sivananda
Rishikesh, India

CONTENTS

PART VI

FINAL VICTORY:

EPILOGUE:

APPENDIX

ABOUT THE AUTHOR

FOREWORD

Dr. Jeanne A. Sloan, DPA
Director of Educational Services
Martin Memorial Hospital
Stuart, Florida 33457

This is the story of an incredibly brave woman who, with the help of her mother, takes on the responsibility of caring for her father after his massive stroke. Afflicted with right-sided paralysis and aphasia (loss of speech and language), Bob Thurston is isolated and terrified in a world where he can neither walk, talk, listen, read, write, dress, or feed himself.

Overcome by fits of depression and rage at his helplessness and inability to communicate, he is at times ignorant of the meaning of words, and unable to recognize his wife or daughter.

The author describes with poignancy and candor the effects of stroke upon the primary caregivers. The same terror, depression, frustration, and anger that envelops the patient are reflected in the lives of the mother and daughter as the catastrophic trauma and devastation of stroke causes illness and collapse of the family structure. Changes in life patterns are produced and roles become reversed. The wife assumes the mother's role, the father becomes the belligerent child, and the daughter assumes the father's responsibilities. Strains are severe and the family becomes desperate for help.

On-the-spot drawings of her father's painfully slow progress bring this journal to life as we follow his rehabilitation through physiotherapy and speech exercises with the help of Home Health. Unfortunately, her mother's health deteriorates due to stress and exhaustion and Doris is burdened with two patients.

Determined to regain her own sanity, she makes several desperate decisions which help her to rise above the "victim" role, eventually helping the family attain some sense of stability.

Medical professionals can benefit from "A Daughter's Story" as the emotional and psychosocial needs of stroke victims are clearly defined. Unless the family actively seeks help and knows where to turn for answers, the health, happiness and successful readjustment to stroke will be sadly lacking.

This is a dramatic story of a family in distress, a handbook for the families of victims of stroke and other catastrophic illnesses and a book of inspiration.

Author's Introduction

This book is offered as a tribute to all the families, wives, husbands, sons and daughters who suddenly find themselves keeper-aide, supporter-companion, guardian, or self-styled prisoner to a stroke victim. When Dad fell ill, I searched the bookstores and library for information which would answer my questions, such as:

1. Will Dad ever walk again?
2. How long does paralysis last?
3. Why is he so depressed?
4. Can he understand me? If so, how well?
5. What's best for the patient—home-care or a nursing home?
6. What is our next step? To whom can we turn?

There was little information at the time. I finally ordered two books on stroke and tried to draw my own conclusions. I decided that first morning, however, that I would keep a record and write my own book about our experience with stroke, in order to help others through similar trying periods.

Dad died five years later, one month after I discovered a stroke club in town. As time mends the wounds of death, I can still cry, but now I cry more for all victims and their families facing the trauma of stroke and caught in the exasperating relationship of caretaker-child or parent-patient. So often the roles become reversed. In our case the parent became the child, the wife became the mother, and the child became the parent.

Dad's illness was a great shock, which ultimately turned into a challenge. As a single woman with professional interests in the arts, I had never raised a family. But my parents became my children. Among other things, I had to hire and fire, solve household problems, learn to keep accounts and repair appliances.

Mother and I had a war going on—a power play, for as she struggled to help Dad, I struggled to let him help himself. As she baby-talked, coddled and pitied him, I reprimanded her for being too kind, dulling his motivation and attempts to be independent. Her great love for him was his cross and his sustenance. It was also the cause of many blow-ups among the three of us.

But let the book speak. And if I share my anguish, my terror and frustration, my aloneness and desperation, I know that I am speaking for many readers who have lived these pages, or who are about to.

I was fifty-two then. Now I am older—but richer perhaps, more compassionate. I have helped to build two stroke clubs, which were desperately needed and unavailable to us. I had no one to cry to, no one to share with who understood. I needed a veteran, someone to let me know that I was not alone—someone who had been there before, who knew what to expect and what to do.

That is the value of a Stroke Club, for we share our problems, our needs, and our successes. That is the value of friends. That is the value of books. May this book become your friend.

Doris Thurston
Stuart, Florida

PART ONE

Struck Down

(March 30, 1876—April 21, 1976)

I

HIS LAST PRUNING

March 30, 1976

The phone rang sharply at 5 a.m.

"Doris, can you come to the hospital right away? Dad had a slight … stroke?" Mother's voice, choked with tears, brought icy fear.

"I'll be right over." I dressed hurriedly in the dark. So this is it, I thought. Dad is seventy-nine. I had often wondered who would go first, and with what illness. I knew that I would be the one to care for them, as my brother, Bob, was married and living in Houston. His two sons were studying to be doctors. My youngest brother, Don, a professor of political science at Union College, New York, was involved in teaching, studying and writing.

That left me, yoga teacher, portrait painter, and occasional entertainer. Still single, my schedule could easily be rearranged to fit my parents' needs. I knew my life would be different from now on. Arriving at the hospital I found Mother seated in a tiny end room dressed in her old green slacks, white curls askew and anxiety in her limpid blue eyes.

"Dad fell on the bathroom floor," she informed me. "We had to wait forty-five minutes for the ambulance."

Dad was groaning in bed and breathing fast. "What time is it?" he asked impatiently.

"It's 5:30 in the morning, Dad. You're in the hospital. Everything's going to be all right," I murmured. I sat in a belated stupor. Was this fragile gentleman with the high, balding forehead and wispy mustache my father? A diagonal scar from an old accident formed a deep crevice across his brow. At twenty-nine, he had collided with a freight train while riding a motorcycle. I often wondered if this blow had not dulled his sense of compassion, for Dad was run by the clock. Every action demanded its precise time and every object its precise place, or there were severe repercussions. I resented this emphasis on organization, perhaps because I felt his need for order took priority over any love he might feel for his wife and children.

Observing his tears of frustration, I was surprised at this sign of vulnerability. His children looked upon him as a tower of strength, a strict disciplinarian, and a person to whom we could always turn for answers. I had seen him cry only twice before, once recently at the death of his sister, and years ago during World War II, when I was attending Syracuse University as a painting student.

I had come home for Easter to seek Dad's guidance. My classmates were being drafted and they were among the new recruits marching beneath the windows of Crouse Hall as we struggled to paint a nude. I was seriously considering joining the Women's Army Corps.

Standing in the rock garden behind our home in Chappaqua, New York, I searched for the correct words. 'Dad, you have given me two years of college and I'm grateful." I always thought my two brothers should go to college, but not me. I had been only six years old when the stock market crashed in 1929 and my memories were still vivid. Dad had been so strapped for money, Mom told me, that he had nearly committed suicide.

"But," I blurted, "I'm thinking about joining the army. Our country is fighting a war and I want to participate. An artist needs to experience life in order to paint, and I could work as occupational therapy assistant in army hospitals, helping returning veterans to recuperate. Besides," I added, "I could earn two more years of education with the GI. Bill. What do you think?"

Dad had been trimming the white roses. He stopped pruning and looked me in the eye.

"It's your decision, Doris. I won't stand in your way. I would be in Iran by now if it weren't for my family. The Texas Company asked me to build asphalt runways for the airfields, but I couldn't leave you three children."

He placed a gloved hand on my shoulder in a rare moment of intimacy. "I love my country, too." His voice broke as tears of frustration welled in his eyes. It was strange to see my father cry and I decided at that moment that I would join the army for *him*. I would do what he could not do. As the oldest child I was free to help my country. My brothers were too young to fight.

My thoughts returned to the present and I looked at him now, aging and helpless. Mother's voice broke into my reverie. "He was pruning the palm trees yesterday. It was too much for him, I guess, but you can't tell him anything." Her mind jumped ahead. "Now I'm afraid we will have to sell the house." She might have been thinking it would be too much for her to handle alone.

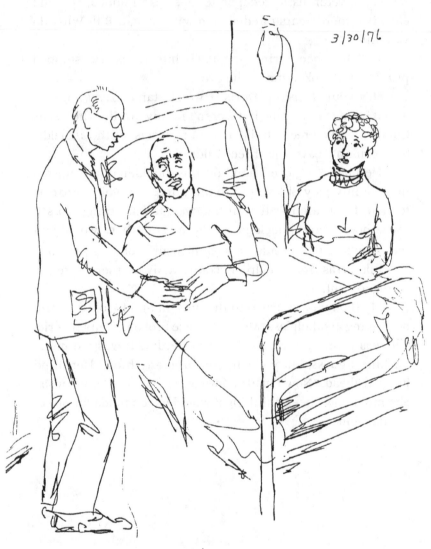

3/30/76

Hospital Visit

Four hours later, the doctor arrived, sauntering into the room with his early-morning-rounds smile. A slight man with an oblique sense of humor, he checked Dad's heart and blood pressure, then hammered his knees and pricked his feet with a pin to check the reflexes.

"You've had a slight stroke, Bob," he announced. "Your mouth is crooked and your thoughts come slower, but you'll pull through and be up and about if you take it easy. You can get up and sit in a chair. Try urinating standing up, but you'll need two people to help you. Can you tell me who is president?"

Dad's mouth twisted into a slow, wry grin. "That's easy—Ford."

"Good! Now, can you say rubber-buggy-bumper?" Dad raised one eyebrow and then struggled with the phrase. "Rubber-bumper."

"Fine," laughed the doctor. "Keep up the good work and you'll be able to go on that cruise you planned to take in the spring."

MASSIVE STROKE

March 1, 1976

My friend, Cheryl, a licensed practical nurse (LPN), called from the hospital about 11 p.m. She had volunteered to sit with Dad while Mother and I got some sleep.

"Doris, your father fell in my arms as I was taking him to the bathroom."

"What do you mean?" I asked in trepidation.

"I'm afraid he's had a massive stroke," she blurted in anguish. "His right arm and leg are completely paralyzed." Energy drained from my body and fear filled my chest. Cheryl was crying now as she added the most devastating news, "And Doris, he can't talk."

"Oh, God, no!" I knew now who would go first. There was nothing for me to do but to help care for him, eventually confronting the enemy—death. I thought of the many times my parents had come to my aid when I was sick or out of a job. They rescued me with love, money, or words of consolation and hope. Now they would be needing me.

I hung up the phone, stunned by the news and numb with fatigue from three exhausting days at the hospital. Appalled at Dad's predicament, I knew I had to do something for the man upon whose wisdom I had always depended, a man who had helped me make decisions, a man whose love I had tried to earn. He was now lying in a hospital bed, paralyzed, speechless, and unable to ring for a nurse. Cheryl would be leaving shortly and I knew what I must do.

Grabbing a blanket and pillow, I drove to the hospital and slipped past the nurse's station. Dad was strapped to the bed with a harness (called a "posy"). The side rails were up and his dark eyes were hollow with fear. Every few seconds he lifted his head to stare at me, dazed and quizzical. "Where am I?" he seemed to be asking. "What are you doing here?"

The room was hot and stuffy because of a broken air conditioner. I opened the window so Dad could breathe, then lay my blanket on the floor to sleep. A nurse bustled in and reprimanded me harshly. She jammed the window shut, then left abruptly.

Suddenly Dad struggled to get out of bed and I tried to restrain him. He fought furiously, gasping for air and roaring like a caged lion. As I rang for the night nurse, it dawned on me. He wanted the urinal. I groped for the plastic bottle, but it was too late.

A tall, capable attendant arrived. I watched, fascinated as he changed the sheets and dressed Dad in a clean hospital gown. I must observe this for future use, I thought. Turning Dad on his side, he rolled the wet sheet close to his body, then turned him back over, removing the sheet. The same procedure was used to insert a clean sheet. When he left, all was quiet, except for the agonized breathing of my patient as he writhed against his bonds.

Lying there at Dad's feet, I had the strange, cold fear that he might die tonight and I would never really have known him. A silent, meditative man, he had been more than my father. He was my teacher and friend. Suddenly the roles were reversed and I had become his guardian.

As my heart contracted in anguish, I had a strange experience: I felt a tall shaft of light hovering over the white-sheathed figure. Beside it, another pillar of light was nudging it and saying, "Move over. I have to fill this area."

The vision passed and Dad didn't die. The next morning, a nurse commended me for staying with him. Mother appeared and we decided to alternate our watches—taking turns feeding him, elevating the bed, fetching water, emptying the urinal and pulling the curtains. The doctor urged us to go home that night as he felt Dad would sleep better without us. I went home and tried to sleep.

It was no use. At 11 p.m., I drove back to the hospital. The nurse was relieved to see me. She had been trying desperately to find a private duty nurse for Dad. As I volunteered my services, Mother appeared. Plopping down a folded blue blanket on the floor beside his bed, she declared: "I'm here. I'll stay."

I left. The next morning, Mother was subdued. It had taken that hectic night for her to realize Dad's true condition. We must keep praying and seeing him whole.

VICTIM

Raging man

    caged,

        speechless,

            in a

hospital bed.

What is left of your former

        self ...

unspeakable majesty ...

          against

the universe.

The will to live is strong

        in this

    man's feeble frame

quick breath of life

    a lovely flame

        pursues

death.

No more my father,

        this

short-seasoned bleat,

he lives

in small time's

tracing.

The silent night

enfolds

us

in one embrace.

I see your former

face.

FLEEING THE TERROR

April 3, 1976

We ordered a cot today and Mother, Cheryl and I will alternate watches. Cheryl gave Dad a bath and shave. Although the nurses have been kind to Dad, they change shifts so often that I feel there is no particular person concerned with his progress. It makes me feel alone in a monstrous impersonal machine. The responsibility lies entirely with us.

Tonight, after being on duty from 4 to 11 p.m., I nearly lost my sanity and sense of self. While sitting with Dad the horror of his condition enveloped me. Crippled and unable to talk or feed himself, he was little more than a vegetable. I absorbed his fear and terror into my own body. My arms became immobile and I felt an insidious paralysis creeping over me, threatening to stop my breath, my life. I had to get away to shake the feeling of death pursuing me. When Cheryl arrived I rushed past her, mumbling, "I've got to get OUT of here!"

Wandering behind the hospital, I sought consolation in a moonlight walk along the river. As I watched little white waves lap at the shore, and stared at the strange sprawling trees silhouetted against the water, I reflected on the mystery of life.

Water. Oceans and rivers teach us how to live, I thought. Water purifies, giving joy and the knowledge that life is continuous—eternal perhaps. And time will be washed away. Whatever problems we have are inconsequential, for this body is not the truth, but only a vessel we travel in to learn the truth. Truth harbors in certain bodies and forms for a little while only.

FIRST COMMUNICATION

April 5, 1976

I am so tired. Mom, Cheryl and I are fighting about who will stay here and when. Life boils down to: "Get the liquids in him ... get out the food ... he's had no B.M. for seven days now ... turn him on his side so he doesn't get any bed burns ...." And, "What in heaven's name does he mean by that gesture?" Dad wiggles his fingers on his good left hand to let us know when he wants to "tinkle." He jiggles the foot of his bed to tell us he wants to sit up higher.

No one seems to know his true condition. Cheryl told me she heard a doctor mutter sadly, "It's too bad. He would have been better off dead." God, it's like riding the crest of a wave, not knowing when or how you'll fall.

ARE MIRACLES POSSIBLE?

10 p.m.

I could not sleep worrying about Dad. I got up and drove to the hospital again. How barren a town can become when one is focused upon a loved one who is ill. Life stops while you wait for death.

Dad was alert and began to make "Wa-wa" sounds, but I couldn't understand what he wanted. He grabbed my arm roughly and turned my body around three times, pointing towards the lights on the river.

"Beautiful, isn't it." I said, hoping that's what he meant. His cries persisted, however. In desperation I rang for the nurse. A buxom black woman and a frail blonde appeared.

"Oh, he wants to sit up," the blonde gushed. Dad nodded in relief. They lifted up the scrawny body, moving him around like a sack of wheat, and gently lowered him into an easy chair. I followed with the glucose bottle held high. They harnessed him to the chair, fluffed a pillow behind his head and left.

"What do I do now?" I wondered, kneeling to massage his foot. He pulled at the vest-like harness that held him prisoner.

"No, I can't untie you, Dad. You might fall." I opened the Bible to "John" and began to read about miracles. Dad's eyes were closed but I knew he was listening. I must remember that "All things are possible with God."

"I DON'T WANT TO DIE!"

April 6, 1976

I am barely alive. After sleeping twelve hours to try and ward off the flu, I woke from a dream in which I was telling my friends, "My Daddy had a stroke! My Daddy had a stroke!" I could see them wince and feel their surge of compassion. But did they know what it really meant?

Dad is closer to the power of God. He is more aware of the breath of life that sustains him moment by moment. He is conscious of pain and numbness in the broken, useless part of his body, but he is awake to the power of food, love, thought, and the healing power of sleep. He is keenly appreciative of the beauty of morning, the sparkling of the river, the wind in the trees and the rhythm of life; the intake and outgo of food and fluid; the blood running like a river through his veins, arteries and heart . . . The river of consciousness. And after it stops at the dam, what then? He is aware, perhaps, that the body drops like a crisp, fallen leaf and the soul goes on. But the seed—the root sprouts. The soul finds a new home and proceeds to grow as the tree re-seeds itself.

Does he believe in reincarnation? Has he a fear of death? "I don't want to die yet. I won't!" I am sure he feels like this, for he is a fighter.

Mother has Dad TRANSFERRED to a beautiful "Room with a view" on the fourth floor. I watch carefully as two nurses wash him. I may have to do this one day - or for several years! little - do I KNOW!

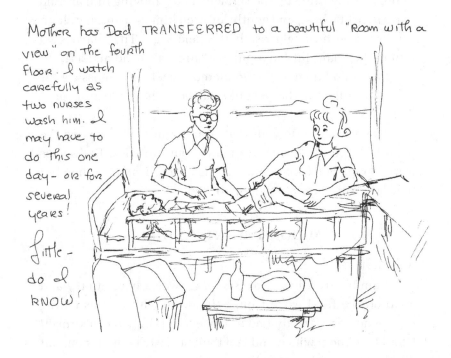

ROOM WITH A VIEW

Letter to my Brothers

April 7, 1976

Dear Bob and Don,

This is a harrowing, heart-rending experience, as majestic and fearful and awesome as birth and death. The beautiful, pitiful in-between time ... the twilight zone between day and night.

I still can't believe it. Dad's stroke is like a wound I carry in my body, or an arm that won't work. But everyday I become more acclimated. Every hour of each new day I try to believe it is real.

I sit in a lovely spacious end room overlooking the St. Lucie River. It is the third and nicest room Mother has claimed for Dad. The day is cloudy. I watch the wind in the palm trees. Every branch that blows seems to be for Dad.

He is resting peacefully after breakfast. I had to feed him. The mouth is twisted down an inch to the left and he can't find his mouth with the spoon. I believe it must feel numb, like his arm and leg. He is motionless and mute—like a huge oak tree with an ax in its side, ready to topple over or grow on for twenty more years.

I feel he is being pruned as he pruned his plants. He loved his rivers and trees so much. Dad still has fight in him, although he is disgusted and can't understand the paralyzed arm. His brain is slowed way down I believe. We must ask pointed questions to get a nod for "Yes" or a shake of the head for "No." Sometimes he doesn't comprehend the difference between yes and no and we have to guess at the answer.

Mother has lost her husband and in his place she finds this stranger. The nasty little remarks he used to make, resented then, would be cherished now. How she misses the caustic lift of the brows, the pursed lips or burning stare. The eyes are mostly vacuous. Occasionally they hold some recognition, although more often, they exude a sick dazed look as he is in and out of sleep. We wonder if he will pull through or become a long-term invalid. This experience has become a nightmarish lesson in death, for our Father takes us home to Himself. I've been through hell thinking, "He'll never make it."

I just talked with a nurse who said, "Keep up the positive thoughts. If he thinks you want him well, it helps. He hears everything. He senses more than you think."

They took a brain scan today to check for damage or for tumors. I'm learning about nursing: bathing, feeding, lifting and physiotherapy. Dad gets very little of that here and no speech therapy.

We must pray.

Love, Doris

MOTHER BREAKS DOWN

April 8, 1976

The strain placed upon both the caregivers and the patient is incredible. Nine days have passed. I have slept here many nights because Dad still can't ring a bell for the nurse. I'm reading *Stroke: The Condition and the Patient* by John E. Sarno, M.D., and Martha Taylor Sarno (McGraw Hill). The book is excellent, posing and answering many questions which might be asked by the stroke victim's family. "A person can stave off a stroke by giving up smoking and drinking, and by changing his diet," Sarno says. How often have we listened to Dad's hacking cough every morning before breakfast after his first cigarette?

I have cried about Dad almost every day, but Mother never broke down until last Sunday. A lovely lady stopped by to pray with her and she finally cried. She still doesn't know who the woman was.

Dad cries a lot. For a man who had little or no patience and showed no emotion, he certainly has changed. All the emotions Dad has repressed are now being released through anger or tears. He always had to do everything himself, but now he must be waited on hand and foot. I feel God has a meaning and purpose behind everything that happens. God is giving me a chance to serve, Mother a greater sense of independence, and Dad a chance to learn patience.

He is irascible at times, yet it's heartening to see him raise both eyebrows or turn his head to signify "no," while giving what might pass for a half smile.

Tonight he actually grasped the spoon and found his mouth. He can use the urinal himself, as long as the nurses or aides remember to put it within reach. His mouth still droops a little, but not so much that it disturbs his good looks. The dull, animal look is gradually disappearing. The doctors tell us he understands almost everything we say.

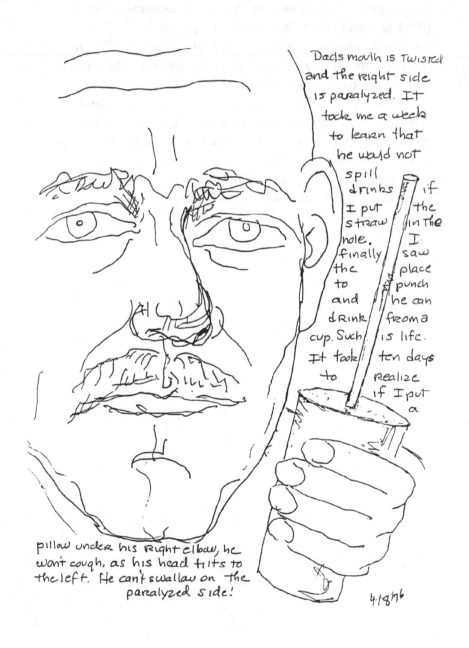

Dads mouth is Twisted and the right side is paralyzed. It took me a week to learn that he would not spill drinks if I put the straw in the hole. I finally saw the place to punch and he can drink from a cup. Such is life. It took ten days to realize if I put a

pillow under his right elbow, he won't cough, as his head tilts to the left. He can't swallow on the paralyzed side!

4/8/76

HOPE OF RECOVERY

April 9, 1976

We have been waiting since Friday for the results of the tests. There is hope for recovery now, at least enough so that Dad will be able to get around with the aid of a walker. I'm betting on it 100 %, although the upper portion of his brain is blocked off by a ruptured artery above the "circle of willis." It could be ten years or more before another stroke carries him away.

This is a learning experience for us all. I want Mom to live long enough to see Dad enjoy life again. He is a fighter and has a desire to live.

Now he appears dazed and in a stupor. He says yes to everything with a nod of his head.

There is often a personality change following a stroke. Medical professionals say that if a person has been nasty and mean in life, he will become docile when he has a stroke. We shall see. Dad was something of a tyrant in my book.

Life is still beautiful. I thank God I live close enough to be able to help. We should send energy and loving thoughts. When I pray for him, I envision the power, starting in his toes and going up the foot and into the leg. The arm will be last, the doctor says, and Dad may never use his hand again.

COMING OUT PARTY

We had a "coming-out party" tonight. After seven or eight days, Dad finally achieved a bowel movement while a sitter was doing just that ... sitting.

I walked into a dark room and found a young man we had hired to look after Dad sitting in a chair while Dad was making sounds like a crazed animal and wildly flailing his arms. There was something on his fingers I thought was blood and I frantically flipped on the light. It was excrement.

"Why didn't you do something?" I asked the paralyzed sitter. "I thought he was crazy," the young man replied. I spent the rest of the evening training the sitter.

The nurses have taken to calling Dad "Houdini" because he gets out of the safety harness when he's sitting down. So far he hasn't been able to get out of it while he's in bed, but he tries and we have to watch him closely.

The physiotherapist is teaching me some exercises, which I help Dad with several times a day. "If we don't do them," he warns, "the tendons in his right arm and leg will shorten and become painful and stiff." Steps in treatment are: 1) Passive movement: (the therapist moves the arm or leg); 2) Active assisted movements: (the patient helps); 3) Active unassisted movements (the patient does the movements).

SECOND MIRACLE

April 10, 1976

When God knocks us down, he creates little miracles to help pick us up. Our first miracle was Cheryl. Little did I expect that she would become so invaluable! She willingly helped out at the hospital and became a steadying influence on us all.

A young woman in her twenties, she took a yoga class with me in my home several months ago. She then called on me and begged to rent the back of my house. Working as a licensed practical nurse with a man who had no legs, she was unhappy with her situation and thought yoga and meditation might bring her peace of mind. I didn't want to rent, but felt that her need was greater than my desire and God might be using me as an instrument. I agreed, and she moved in.

Our second miracle occurred today. Blind with fatigue, I called on a neighbor I knew slightly through a yoga class to ask if she would sit with Dad. She wasn't home but I described my problem to her brother, Nelson, who had just arrived in Florida. He was a pale-faced youth with a shock of black wavy hair and a limp due to a bad knee.

"My sister won't be able to help you, but I'll be glad to," he said eagerly. "I'm a licensed practical nurse and a stroke-aide specialist. I love to help stroke patients walk again." He promised to visit Dad at the hospital.

MINOR SUCCESSES

April 11, 1976

"He rang for me last night," a nurse told me when I arrived at the hospital this morning. I was ecstatic. That small triumph meant he could be more independent and we could get more sleep at night. I had painted the call bulb fluorescent orange so he could find it easier at night and wondered if this had helped.

The doctor examined him today and reported that nerves in his foot, which had been totally unresponsive, had regained some function. Great! He said that an EEG demonstrated that seventy-five percent of Dad's brain is working and he can understand everything we say, even if we can't always understand him. With persistent therapy, the doctor said, he might regain the use of his arm and leg.

"He's not feeling well," Mother whispered to me later and I took her aside. "Let's try not to make any negative statements in his presence. Now that we know he can understand us, let's say only affirmations. If we picture him healthy, happy and strong, he'll become that."

I worked with Dad using some acupressure techniques I had read about and was giving him some physiotherapy when Nelson arrived. He taught me a new exercise, showing me how to lift Dad's knee and flex the foot while getting Dad to push against my shoulder. Mother decided to hire the hospital physiotherapist once a day. Medicare will pay eighty-five per cent of the cost.

Dad was disturbed today. Whenever Mother and I are in his room together he gets confused and upset because we argue and interrupt each other, rather than speaking slowly one at a time. We *must* work harder to remain calm and positive around him.

A social service worker suggested that we check into getting a biofeedback machine that gives an audible beep when a muscle is working, but mother wasn't interested. A nurse advised us to do whatever we can to stimulate all of Dad's senses—sight, smell, hearing, touch and taste. I plan to bring in a mirror so he can watch himself eat. Perhaps then he won't spill as much.

Nelson brought in a ball today and had Dad squeeze it with his good left hand. Then he put the ball into his paralyzed right hand and said, "Squeeze. You must do this." But Dad wasn't able to.

We can no longer leave the bed raised and walk out, as Dad is no longer in the safety harness.

This
nuRse
was
delightful,
and The
only one
slightly
HUMAN,
She
actually
woRe a
smile—
and
was
good
enough
to look
up The
pill
Dad was
being given—
though This
is against
the
RULES!

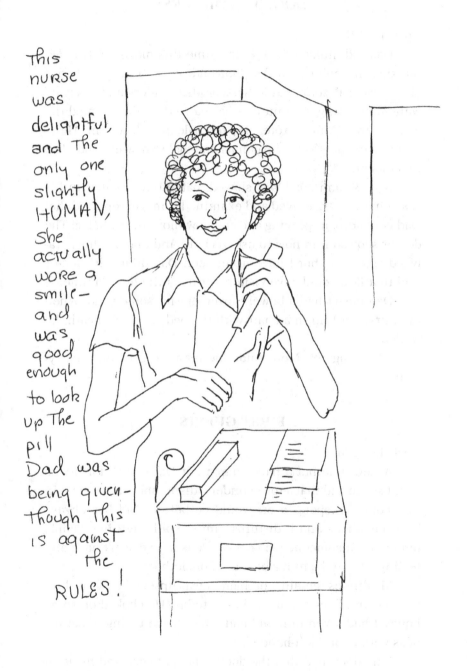

DOCTOR'S ORDERS!

April 12, 1976

Dad fed himself for the first time this morning. Hurray! But then he pointed to the floor and began a raucous series of "Wa-wa-wa" sounds. Mother couldn't understand what he wanted and rang for a nurse who realized that he wanted the bed lowered. Mom wrote, "He fell asleep at 8:20 a.m. He is wearing his new yellow pajamas and looks so sweet and alert this morning."

By 9:30 a.m. Dad was shaved, bathed and seated in his easy chair. Dr. P. arrived and examined him. He reported that Dad is steadily improving and can now move his right leg. The doctor showed him how to use his left hand to move his paralyzed right one, but I have never seen Dad do it. The doctor said that Dad could have visitors for five minutes at a time.

Dad hasn't had a bowel movement for some time. When the nurse sat him in a chair with the bedpan underneath, he wailed.

"Never again," Mom said. She plans to get him a potty-chair.

FIRST GUESTS

April 13, 1976

A new aide put a paper napkin at Dad's neck for breakfast. I suggested that a towel under a disposable plastic napkin that could be sponged off would be better. Dad has always been fastidious and it disturbs him to spill anything. People tend to treat someone who can't talk as if he doesn't have any feelings. I'll make him a bib out of oilcloth.

Mealtimes remain a problem. I was upset when I saw him try to drink from the urine bottle today. He choked on some honey I had given him and had a hard time trying to eat his peas with a fork, left-handed.

I'm concerned that the doctor has put eggs and meat on

his diet. My yoga guru, Swami Vishnu DeVenanda, author of *The Complete and Illustrated Book of Yoga,* teaches that meat and animal products such as milk, cheese and eggs cause high blood pressure and hardening of the arteries. It is a proven fact that as weight rises, so does blood pressure. Less salt is better. One can use lemon juice and spices when cooking veggies and substitute yogurt for sour cream on salads.

Two friends arrived at 2:30 pm. After a few minutes, Dad became very emotional, crying and pointing wildly towards the desk. We couldn't understand what he was trying to tell us. Our minister arrived and solved the mystery: Dad was pointing at the clock, apparently demanding that his guests adhere to the doctor's five-minute dictum. Promptness has always been one of his attributes.

DON IS COMING

April 14, 1976

I lay on my altar rug Sunday night, trying to be used as a channel of healing power for Dad. Cheryl meditated with me. As she helps us, we are helping her. "My need is your fulfillment."

Last night, a nurse told me that Dad is a flirt and everyone loves him. He still can't speak. When he tries, he manages only to say "Wa-wa-wa." I don't know whether he should be starting speech lessons, or whether it will simply come.

Today I am hopeful, but sometimes I feel so gloomy that I find it difficult to write. I'm up and down. But Cheryl says stroke patients themselves are up and down and we can only pray to God for power, peace and the wisdom to cope with whatever He gives us. And try to see Dad whole.

I am taking a Dale Carnegie class and it is very good therapy for spouses and caregivers. In it I learn: "What a man can conceive and believe, a man can achieve."

I told a nurse of my concern about Dad's diet and she confirmed that a low cholesterol diet is good for stroke and heart patients. In *"Stroke: The Condition and the Patient,"* John and Martha Taylor Sarno write: "Cholesterol crystals are deposited in the walls of arteries, increasing in number and size until a blood clot forms and occludes the artery and a rupture occurs." My brother, Don, arrived for a visit tonight and it was a very emotional scene. Dad shed tears of joy when he saw him. I myself had wept when I first heard he was coming. It will be great to have some support.

GETTING OUT OF BED

April 15, 1976

"Today Bob looks alert and well," Cheryl reported. "He is eating alone, seated in his easy chair. I talked about my day. He understood every word. I encouraged him to lift the bad leg by using the strong one underneath, when getting out of bed. At first he refused to cooperate. Then he did it and laughed. This is very helpful in getting him back to bed also."

TRAPEZE

April 16, 1976

Don and I bought a trapeze for Dad's bed today. When it came time for Mother to feed him dinner, I showed him how to grab the trapeze with his left hand and pull himself up. He couldn't do it and protested loudly.

"Dad, you can help me," I scolded. "I know how we can do it. We don't need two nurses to get you higher. Now use your good leg to push yourself up higher and pull with your good arm." He did.

I discovered today that by placing a pillow under the paralyzed arm, the body tilts to the left. Now when Dad swallows, he won't choke so much on the paralyzed side. I tried to teach Dad yoga breathing in the hope that the increased flow of oxygen would help him recover.

"Relax, Dad. Breathe through the nose and fill your abdomen like a balloon," I instructed. He breathed through his mouth, but he did take a few longer, deeper breaths. It's difficult to know how much he understands.

"Breathing deeply will bring oxygen to the brain and help to heal you," I explained slowly. He began to cooperate. "As a yoga teacher," I continued, "I know the value of oxygen or 'prana,' which is the life source. Breathing deeply is like watering plants, feeding all your muscles, tissues and organs with energy and new life." I thought of the many times this exercise had helped to keep me from falling asleep while driving, possibly even saving my life. Perhaps it could help wake up some inactive cells in Dad's brain.

Just as yoga exercises and deep breathing affect organs and glands, so, too, does acupressure massage stimulate the endocrine system. I am working on Dad's big toe, circling and pressing the points for the pituitary gland and the pineal. The pituitary is the master gland and helps to balance all of the other glands, including the adrenals, thyroid and sex glands.

Dad's spine is crooked and one leg is three inches higher than the other. I'd like to take him to a chiropractor, but Mother will not hear of it. I'm not sure Dad would cooperate, anyway.

ART THERAPY

April 17, 1976
    I gave Dad a pencil and pad today as part of an "art lesson." As we started, I realized I didn't have my glasses. He laughed and gestured for me to borrow his, then drew three spirals with his left hand.

"Good," I said. "The evoluting circle symbolizes life. Now, let's draw a sun." I drew a circle and added spokes. His pencil froze and he started to cry in frustration.

"Don't worry. You'll learn," 1 assured him. "We have to retrain the brain how to use the left hand." Slowly and meticulously he copied over my drawing. I sketched three tiny circles and he duplicated them. Then he drew two circles, connected them and added tails.

"Glasses?" I asked in surprise.

EASTER HOPE

April 18, 1976

I arrived at Dad's spacious corner room this Easter morning. Plants lined the windowsill and the curtains were closed. My father was raving in his guttural "Ah-ah-ahs," and pointing to the curtains. I opened them, but he raved even more vigorously. I closed them again and, on impulse, I put a little plant in the crook of his good left arm.

His cries stopped abruptly and our eyes locked. Never before in our fifty-three years together had we seemed to be so truly aware of each other. The moment contained knowledge of the immediacy of life and the dreadful finality of death,

His glance dropped to the little plant and he pressed the dry earth with his good index finger. The gesture contained a lifetime of love for nature. In that moment I loved him deeply. He looked up and a torrent of tears flooded his face as the room echoed with his sobs. I thought of the contrast between his present self and the silent reserved man my father had been—undemonstrative, void of all emotion except when he was cutting us down. Awareness of the torment of his present life washed over me, and my own tears began to flow.

"Dad," I pleaded "This plant is like our lives. We have only a limited time here on earth, then we wilt and die. You nearly went, but you didn't. You need water; we all need water. God is trying to teach us a lesson. You'll see. We have to go into the dark to see the light."

I placed the plant on the windowsill. Three nurses arrived to transport my father to the armchair next to the large picture window. They opened the curtains and we could see one sailboat on a ruffled river in the morning sunlight.

Dad was still crying, his head weaving from side to side

like a luffing sail. The twisted mouth drooped to the right. Easter meant so much to him. He had been a deacon. I thought
he was the handsomest of men as he proudly carried the collection plate forward, head held high. When he returned to sit
with the family I felt the quiet strength of his presence and
wondered what was in his mind.

Now, seeing him in despair, I fell to my knees and clasped
his legs to my chest. "Dad, listen to me," I implored. "Today
is Easter. You and I helped to crucify Christ, but today he is
resurrected. And things happened to the people around him.
It's the same with you. You were struck down, but there is a
beautiful purpose behind it all, don't you see? It's so we can
love each other more in our suffering. We have more growing
to do."

I felt like Mary Magdalene kneeling at the feet of Christ.
The plant was dry; it needed water just as our family needed love and understanding. Dad had always been the ruler,
whittling my mother down with his constant criticism. Now,
over the last few weeks, I had watched her love and devotion
blossom, enveloping this man, who had suddenly become her
child.

My own compassion had been nurtured by the tears of
my pain. As I watered the little plant, I thought about our
lives—how much we do need the water of life to enrich the
love power in our hearts.

DAD'S DEPRESSION

April 19, 1976

Dad is deeply depressed, perhaps because the doctor
plans to release him to a convalescent home tomorrow. I had
wanted to join Mother and Don for dinner tonight, but when
I arrived at the restaurant, Mother was very upset over Dad's
depression.

I decided to pick up Nelson, instead, and we went to the
hospital where we found Dad in low spirits indeed. He waved

his left hand in a gesture of dismissal. He didn't want visitors, nor did he welcome therapy. A nurse bustled in and immediately understood the situation.

"Don't leave, folks. I'll be back in a minute with some ice cream." She turned to my father and said cheerfully, "That ought to make you happy. And don't forget our date?" She winked and Dad's eyebrow flickered in response.

I sat down and opened a Bible. Nelson stood at the foot of the bed where he could watch Dad's response. He spoke directly to me. "I have helped several stroke patients walk again." His voice was purposeful and controlled.

"It takes will power and determination. I believe your father is very persistent. I am quite sure he could learn to walk again because he has what it takes." He paused significantly. "Mr. Thurston has will power!" I looked at Dad. His eyes were closed but I was sure that the words had sunk into his consciousness, perhaps offering a glimmer of hope.

"I don't believe you should put your father into a convalescent home tomorrow," Nelson said as we were driving home. "He is too depressed; it will surely kill him. He'll be able to recuperate better in his own environment. If you let me work with him, I believe I could get him walking again in a month or two."

The darkness seemed to lift. On a sudden hunch, I invited him to come with me to Dad's house in Jensen Beach to see the layout. Don met us at the door and I explained the situation.

"Let him speak to Mother first, so she doesn't feel it's our idea," Don suggested. I agreed. When Mother entered the living room, I noticed how stooped and slight she seemed, too slight, perhaps, to bear such a heavy burden. Nelson began outlining his proposal.

"Mrs. Thurston, I have been observing your husband at the hospital and giving him some physiotherapy. I believe he has a greater chance to improve if you bring him home. He can sit in the sun, friends can visit him and he can exercise every day.

"You would need an aide, of course. As I am a Licensed Practical Nurse (LPN), and have had experience with stroke patients, I would be willing to watch your husband twenty-four hours a day for six days a week. If you give me a thirty-day trial period, I'll even sleep in his room on a cot if you wish, and build ramps for the wheelchair so we can wheel him outdoors."

Mother obviously had mixed feelings about Nelson's proposal. On one hand, she wouldn't have to make the daily wearing nursing home visits. On the other was the fear that total care of an invalid would be too much for her, even with Nelson's help.

I interrupted with a proposal of my own: "Let's pray about it." I led the way into Mother's bedroom and we sat in a circle on her blue rug and prayed aloud for guidance. After a little more discussion, we decided to take Nelson up on his offer. What did we have to lose? Tomorrow we would ask his doctor if we could bring Dad home.

Nelson seemed to glow from within now that he had a purpose. He confided that he had recently lost his young wife to cancer and was very much at loose ends.

"Your husband's need is my need," he said and his brown eyes, so like Dad's, filled briefly with tears. "I'm sure he can walk again—with a lot of hard work."

Do angels come with a limp and curly brown hair?

DOCTOR'S CHOICE

April 20, 1976

Mother called the doctor in the middle of the night to tell him of our decision to take Dad home and he was understandably angry. He ordered us to have Dad out of the hospital by 1 p.m., despite the fact that we had no bed for him yet.

"What would really be best for Dad, the convalescent home or his own home?" I asked.

"He would get better care and more therapy at home," he said. "I think he would deteriorate in the convalescent home." So Nelson was right. I was exhilarated. We must get Dad in a positive mood, make him work, and give him hope—knowing he can do it. And he will do it. Have faith.

FAMILY DECISION

April 21, 1976

The doctor has allowed Dad to stay another day. Don is renting a bed and has ordered a collapsible wheelchair. I massaged Dad's back and leg and gave him acupressure. He cooperated, pushing his paralyzed leg against my hand. Apparently he has some nerve function in his right leg.

Sometimes I think the presence of the family makes Dad feel more depressed and inadequate. We must try to be cheery and not get upset if we can't understand him. This morning he kept pointing to the bathroom door and raving. I couldn't find anything in there and finally closed the door in disgust and rang for the nurse. What will we do when we have no nurse to ring for?

The nurse found two of our empty vases under the bathroom sink. Dad knows we are going home tomorrow and doesn't want to leave anything behind. I look forward to our experience with trepidation, already questioning the validity of our decision. But there is no doubt that Dad has come out of yesterday's depression.

PART TWO

COMING HOME

(April 22, 1976—August 24, 1976)

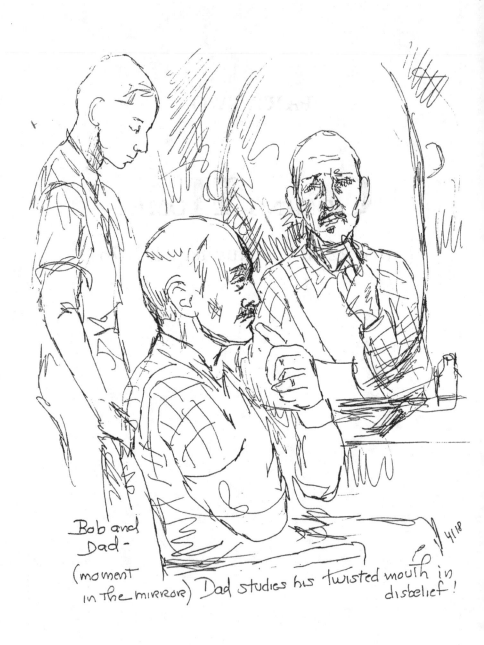

Bob and
Dad -
(moment
in the mirror) Dad studies his twisted mouth in
disbelief!

II

UNEXPECTED VISITOR

April 22, 1976

Dressed in crisp blue pajamas and a maroon robe, Dad was taken home today. Nelson wheeled him into the living room in the new blue wheelchair and Dad smiled a greeting to the white cat guarding the front door.

One of several animals he created in ceramics class a few years ago, she is calm and imperious. This shiny effigy never fails to amuse me, for Dad loves kittens but has little use for grown cats.

Surveying the living room through tears of joy, Dad is obviously glad to be home. Here he can view sparkling blue water and colored clouds, watch sea gulls, hear birds singing, listen to Mother's piano at eventide and hear the train's passing. Nelson and I transferred him to his easy chair next to the grand piano. From here he can view the world as though from the bow of a ship.

To the East, the spacious lawn studded with thirty-eight palm trees slopes towards the river. Sitting on a long, low pine bench under the sliding glass windows, potted plants and assorted birds keep silent company. Dad built the bench in his carpenter shop in the garage. A graceful white heron balancing on one leg bears the initials R.R.T. An owl with tufted ears and a pudgy orange beak, its huge sightless eyes formed by two-indented thumb marks, stands majestic and proud.

Among my gifts to Dad is an elegant mahogany egret, who's curved neck thrusts upwards above slender stalk-like legs. Its squared-off wings are worn like a draped cape. A preposterous pelican with huge shell feet squats beneath the egret, along with three small wooden birds from India, whose hollowed out middles form napkin holders.

Dad's eyes travel to the textured wooden ceiling, which flows from living room to Florida room, creating an indoor-outdoor feeling of space. Aqua curtains alternate with pine-paneled walls, offsetting the soft, green rug. Dad must be proud of this house, I mused, for he designed it himself and built it twenty-five years ago when he came to Florida from Chappaqua. Not until I lived here alone one summer (while my parents took a trip to Europe), did I realize that my father, too, was an artist. Perhaps, from him, I received my aware-ness of line, shape, color and form.

This house reflects his love for the sea. Seated at the "helm" in his worn beige easy chair, he can watch the sun rise in the East and set in the West. Glowing reds, pinks and violets are echoed in the forsythia, azalea and bougainvillea bushes. To the West are three royal palm trees behind slid-ing glass doors, which Dad dubbed "The Trinity." Close by a slender gray section of tree spews from the earth, which I call "The Serpent." Next to the back door is a "Crown-of-Thorns" plant. All this is in a part of Jensen Beach known as "Eden."

Dad has been a loner all his life, keeping his emotions to himself. I never really knew his thoughts about God. Yet, I know how much he loves nature. If he loves God half as much as he loves nature, he must love God a whole lot.

The house feels still and quiet now that Dad is resting. There will be moments, no doubt, when we will wonder if we did the right thing in bringing him home. Dad is to sleep in his hospital bed in the pink guestroom in the back of the house. Nelson will sleep on a cot beside the bed.

After dinner, I stepped into the backyard to watch a flaming red sunset. I was startled to see a screech owl seated on a tree branch. I called Mother to join me and we stood immobile as the owl slowly turned its head to stare at us. Dad howled excitedly from his wheelchair.

Dad is the wise one, I thought, combining the silent inscrutability of his white ceramic cat with the reputed wisdom of the mysterious owl with all-seeing eyes. The owl slowly swiveled his head back to center, indifferent to us.

Later I looked up the entry on owls in our encyclopedia and read part of it aloud to Mother: "The screech owl is a woodland bird. They are the only owls with ear tufts. At night they give their weird trembling calls and hollow whistles which run down the scale. Superstitious persons in the South think these sounds mean that death or disaster is near."

Owls are Dad's favorite birds. Besides his ceramic owl, he has a wooden mobile owl hanging on the front porch and a copper owl with spreading wings in the bookcase. Despite the encyclopedia, I'm inclined to believe that our night visitor is a good omen.

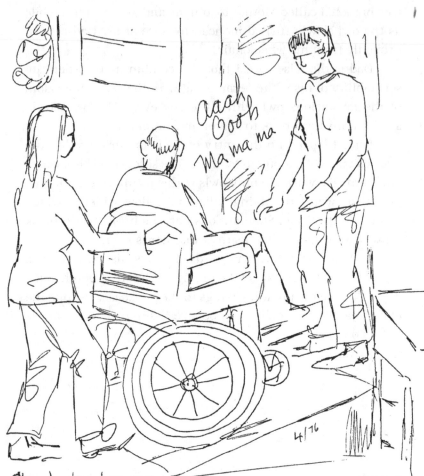

Cheryl teaches me how to take Dad down the ramp BACKWARDS, which is safer! This is Dad's first trip to the "Observation Tower", which is really just our screened in porch, from which he contentedly points out birds, boats and turtles.

PART-TIME HELP

April 23, 1976

Nelson has disappeared. He was obviously exhausted trying to work around the clock. He also had difficulties with
Mom. An experienced aide, he felt he knew what was good
for the patient, but Mother seldom agreed. This leaves me on
night duty. I sleep on the couch in the living room, waking
every time Dad groans or has to use the urinal.

We hired a part-time aide through a local Bible college.
Rose, a lay minister's wife and mother of two small children,
works with us on Saturdays. She bathes and dresses Dad, helps
him exercise and does the cooking and cleaning. Quiet and
shy, she is as gentle and peaceful as a flower. This morning
she moved all the potted plants outside and watered them,
with Dad's supervision.

Despite Rose's assistance, we need full-time help desperately. Today Cheryl surprised me by asking if she could work
for us. "But you have a job already" I protested. She worked as
nurse to a man who has no legs. "I wouldn't want you to leave
your bed-patient. Besides, your boss is a friend of ours."

"My employer understands," she assured me. "I'd much
rather teach a man to walk than work with someone who will
never walk again. I was really hurt that you never considered
me for the job," she confessed. "After I told my boss about my
experience as a stroke patient aide and how much I really
wanted to help your father walk again, she said, 'Go with God.
Go where you are needed!'"

So Cheryl has come back into our lives. As she is renting
a room at my studio in Stuart, we will take different shifts.
Perhaps she will prove more stable than Nelson. But I will
always be grateful to Nelson. After all, he gave us the incen-
tive to bring Dad home and the courage to believe he could
walk again. Sometimes I feel that God is up there pulling the
strings, and all we have to do is to play the game.

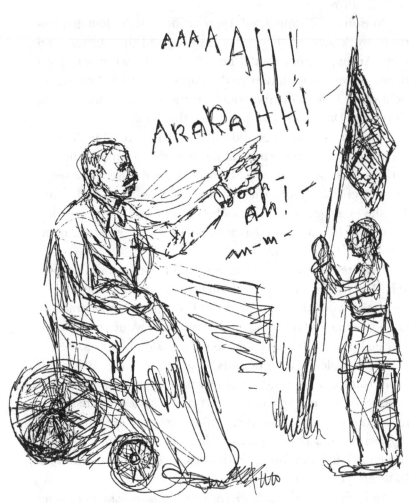

As I struggled to put up the flag, Dad
kept up a tirade of "Ah-h-h's". How can he
be so smart and not talk while I'm so dumb
and can talk?

FLAG RAISING

April 24, 1976

Today is Sunday and I am on duty all day for the first time. I bathed Dad and brought him breakfast in bed. He yelled and pointed to the tray until I finally realized that I had forgotten his prune juice.

This afternoon our friend Ray arrived with 3-D pictures of Dad and Mother before his stroke. This brought a fresh supply of tears. Dad knows that his mouth now droops on the right side. He often sits with his head slumped forward and frequently drools. To divert his attention, Mom came onto the sun porch where we were sitting, an American flag over her arm. "Bob, do you want us to put up the flag?" He nodded yes and as she dropped her end on the ground, I reprimanded, half in jest, "Mother, it's a sin to let the flag touch the ground." Mother walked off in a huff, leaving me to manage the flag alone.

Dad kept up a continual tirade of "Wa-wa-wa's," trying to direct me from the porch. I was filled with childish fears that I would make a major blunder. Sure enough, when I raised the flag, it was upside down. I wondered how Dad could be so smart and not talk, while I could be so stupid and talk.

This last indignity infuriated Dad. Ray came to my rescue and we managed to raise the flag correctly, completing a ritual which had long symbolized to my father his deep love and respect for the country he cherished, and ideals for which he would have fought had he the opportunity.

ON DUTY

April 25, 1976

Cheryl arrived at 7 a.m. and left at 8 p.m. "A very long day," she wrote in the daily journal: "Mr. T looks well this morning. He stayed in bed until after lunch. I put him into the wheelchair at 1:15 p.m. It was too windy to haul the flag up, so we sat in the backyard in the sun. Last night he helped me fold the American flag, which was quite an accomplishment. Today we watched the telephone men work on wires.

"When I wheeled him through the garage, he saw a big spider and ordered me to chase it out. I pushed him around front and he motioned that he wanted the grass cut. Returning to the living room we looked at photographs of the Maine cottage. When Mrs. T. got up from her nap, she kissed him and he began to cry.

"Mr. T is like a baby. I rub his back while he's in the wheelchair and he loves it. Doris, we need a radio for Mr. T. I played mine today while dressing him and he liked it. Now he is crying because I read him a card from Bob. I quickly placed the mirror in front of him and he stopped crying long enough to study his mustache and teeth. Then he laughed. A good way to stop the crying is to sidetrack him." NOTE: J.E. Sarno says in *A Guide for Patients and Their Families* that crying is practically universal after a stroke because the patient's "Cry‗control center" has been temporarily damaged. Laughter and crying are not always appropriate.

"This job is long and tiring." Cheryl continues. "But it will be worth it if we can get him to walk. I miss seeing Doris as our shifts don't overlap. It is hard to believe that a week ago we performed religious dances for the Ministerial Association based on her Beatitude paintings. One never knows what God has in store for us."

REPORT

April 26, 1976

Cheryl's report: "All is perfect here. Your Mom is beautiful and I love her. She gives me much respect and concern. Sunday she was upset with me, but I am beginning to feel at home here now. I always did seek family in strangers. Doris, although I don't see you much, I want you to know that you haven't lost a friend. You've gained a family member. I care.

"I'm also overtired. I'm leaving now. I just put two blankets on 'Dad.' The windows are opened a little. The night-light is on. Today I encouraged him to use hand movements instead of groaning. Remind him that instead of groaning, he can help by putting sounds to movement."

INJURED BIRD

April 27, 1976

I slept in Stuart last night. Awakening early this morning, I found two birds in the street in front of my house. The female was wounded. Her mate, a black and white-winged bird, was trying to move her. As I approached them, he flew away. The poor injured bird was plopped forward on her chest, wings beating. Her eyes kept opening and shutting. I picked up the broken creature and placed her by the side of the road.

"I'm sorry," I murmured. Her broken body reminded me of my stricken father.

After a swim in the ocean, I returned to find both birds gone. I cried. Where do birds go to die? We see them all around us in the fullness of their lives, but seldom see dead or dying birds. I was touched by the male's devotion to his injured mate and it made me consider Mom's even greater love and devotion to Dad. One forgets the magnificent courage, will power, and self sacrifice that animals and humans are capable of, even to the laying down of one life for another.

We must buy a bird feeder to hang under the eaves at the back of the house so that Dad can watch the cardinals, robins and blue jays.

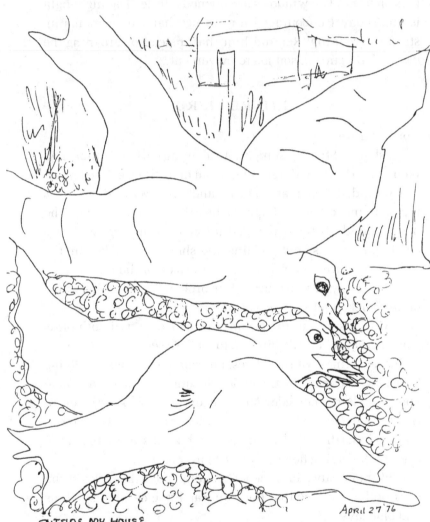

April 27 '76

OUTSIDE MY HOUSE

A Black and white bird had been injured, perhaps by a car. Seeing fluttering wings, I discovered The poor broken body, chest slightly smashed, little eye full of fear. Its friend flew away as I approached. I believe The other bird was trying to help him get out of the Road. I moved the hurt bird and Thought, "For they shall be comforted..."

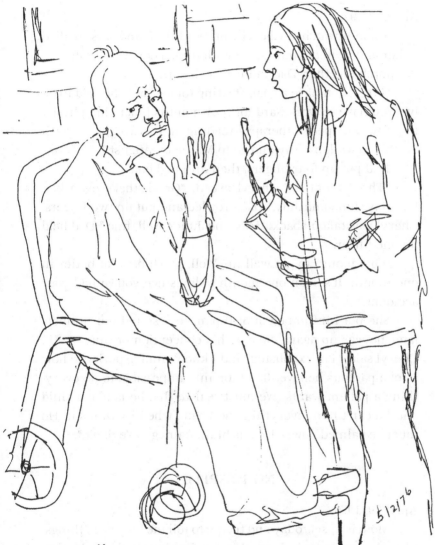

Cheryl: "You have a goal now, Mr. T. Starting tomorrow you must work hard, physiotherapy. Four months! and you'll be able to walk and go to Maine by August." Dad holds up three fingers!

THE GOAL

April 28, 1976

Today I watched Cheryl work with Dad and was thrilled at her ability to communicate with him. They were seated on the porch together, Dad in his wheelchair.

"Mr. T, you have a goal, starting tomorrow," she said firmly. "You have to work hard for four months practicing physiotherapy and speech therapy—reading and writing, and you'll be able to walk by July and go to Maine by August."

Dad put up four fingers, then dropped one.

"Three months?" Cheryl asked. "Good, that's even better. May, June and July." Dad growled and put up two fingers. Cheryl was taken aback. "May and June? Well, fine." Dad held up one finger.

"One month to get well in? Well, you'll be a lot better in one month. It's been one month today since you've had your accident."

She put him to bed at 5:30 p.m. to rest and ten minutes later he was up again. "Maybe his conception of time is off," Cheryl said. "I'm exhausted, and I know from experience how stroke patients behave. It is humanly impossible to do everything a patient wants. We must realize that he is like a child and he can't have everything he wants when he wants it. He must be calmed down. He has brain damage. We don't."

NO RESPITE

April 29, 1976

Mom is upset today and trying to tell me how to do things. Cheryl complained about this on Sunday. Perhaps Mother needs time alone with Dad. She could read him the newspaper or do speech therapy. But it should be in the schedule so he can feel her presence and know it is his time with her. She feels useless and left out if Cheryl and I do everything. After all, she used to live alone with him here and now others are taking over.

It is difficult, however, to work with Dad while Mom is in the room. We argue over which pair of underpants to put on him, what color shirt, which trousers. When we argue, Dad gets extremely upset and tops us both with his raving.

I wish Mom had some friends of her own that she could go out to lunch with, but they all seem to come in couples at cocktail time. Dad likes to see them as long as they don't all talk at once. It's hard for him to understand more than one person at a time.

I have been on duty alone today and learn that this is a very hard job indeed. No wonder Nelson quit and Cheryl gets very tired. There is no respite, as Dad needs constant attention—getting him up and down, tying and untying his sling, buttoning and unbuttoning his sweater, opening and closing doors, taking him to the john and back. Perhaps it's the long hours from 8 a.m. to 8 p.m. which makes this job so difficult.

HOME HEALTH

April 30, 1976

Our third miracle occurred today as a result of meeting a mysterious stranger on a California beach last summer. He and several others were praying for a girl who was an alcoholic and suicidal. I talked with him about yoga, acupressure, reflexology and God.

He knocked on my door this morning after bicycling all the way from California. I gasped, for he looked just like my vision of "John" from the Bible—strong, tall and muscular, with a black beard and an inner beauty. He asked if he could use my studio to hold an acupressure seminar for my friends so that he could earn enough money to bike to Miami.

I called a social worker friend at the hospital. She declined the invitation and asked me about Dad. I told her we had him at home, she suggested that we contact Home Health Services. That was the first I'd heard of it, so my friend filled me in.

"If you contact them within fourteen days of your father's release from the hospital, you will be able to get physiotherapy, speech therapy, a nurse and an aide who will come four hours a day to wash and dress your father. You must have the permission of your doctor, and Medicare will pay for most of it." (Note: Occupational therapy and a psychologist are now available through Medicare.)

I was overjoyed and called Home Health immediately. A Home Health nurse arrived that afternoon to evaluate Dad's case. Wholesome, bouncy, and blonde, Olga was in her late forties with an intriguing Norwegian accent accompanied by an engaging smile. She walked into our hearts and we were only too glad to answer her simple questions: "How old is he? What insurance does he have? When did he retire? When did he have his stroke? What are the results?"

NOTE: All families should be notified of Home Health or Visiting Nurse Services by doctors, nurses, or social workers, before they leave the hospital. Often these services are indispensable, particularly if the caregiver or spouse is ill or exhausted and needs help. If informed, he or she will be able to contact the patient's doctor, tell him her predicament, and he can prescribe assistance.

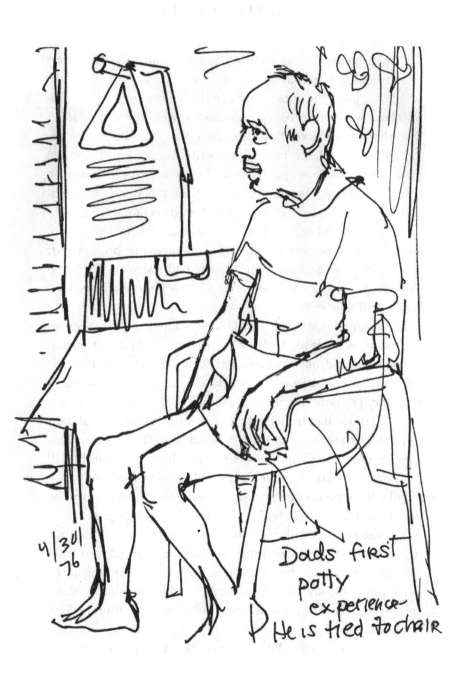

4/30/
76

Dads first
potty
experience
He is tied to chair

ANNABEL ARRIVES

April 31, 1976

Annabel, our new licensed practical nurse (LPN) from Home Health, barreled in forty-five minutes late.

"I vas lost," she apologized in a thick German accent. "The numbers were running up and down every which way and I thought I would never find this house."

Setting her large black bag on the living room floor, she pulled out a stethoscope and marched into Dad's bedroom. A sturdy middle-aged woman with a mellifluous voice, she greeted Dad with a warm handshake and an infectious smile.

"Good morning, Mr. Thurston. Would you like me to take your blood pressure? Good." She wrapped the broken cuff around his arm and went on: "You've had a stroke. The blood clot will dissolve itself. When a blood vessel bursts a new blood vessel will take over."

Invisible layers of fear, like worn-out garments, seemed to drop away from my body as I sensed the determination and purpose behind her brusque, but friendly, manner. Beneath her words I could hear the unspoken message: "Don't waste my time. I'm here to get you walking. Work with me or else!"

The office had informed me that Annabel was one of their top practical nurses and I easily believed it. God is good. This woman will bring hope into our home, hope that surely will be contagious and to which Dad will respond positively. Annabel will come every morning from 8 a.m. to 10 a.m. to bathe and dress Dad. Cheryl will work from 10 a.m. to 7 p.m.

I watched carefully as Annabel gave Dad a bed bath using two bowls. She turned him on his side, washed him from the first bowl, and rinsed him from the second. Starting at the head and neck, she moved down his body. One side washed, she turned him over and washed the other side, then let him wash his own genitals.

"In three weeks, I'll bet you'll be talking and walking

again," she said. Dad winced and cried, slowly shaking his head.

"Don't cry, Mr. T. You are just pitying yourself and that doesn't help," she reprimanded. He continued to cry.

"Mr. T, there is a man I know who lives somewhere around here whom I helped to walk again," Annabel said firmly. "He's over eighty. He improved after doing his exercises, and now he is using a walker."

I had found it difficult to believe that my father would ever walk again. I knew little about stroke and doubted if Dad knew any more. How ghastly to be in his condition and have absolutely no knowledge of strokes, people who had suffered from them and survived, or even learned to walk. I remembered seeing a stroke-aphasic in a movie and being horrified at the man's condition. It must be the worst thing that can happen to a human being, I thought at the time—a living death. Thus Annabel's words were as welcome as a life raft to a drowning man.

"Mr. T, you need patience," she scolded. "Crying won't help. Now, let's see you smile." Annabel's positive manner brought tears of joy to my eyes. Perhaps Dad could learn to walk again. Lying there helpless, paralyzed completely on the right side and unable to talk, it would take bull-headed determination, courage and persistence to act as if he believed he could get well.

With Annabel's vitality and assertive spirit, Dad began to cooperate, trying hard to concentrate upon the stubborn muscles in what appeared to be a dead leg.

"I think I feel a live nerve, Mr. T. Keep up your exercise and I guarantee you will be walking in a month or two."

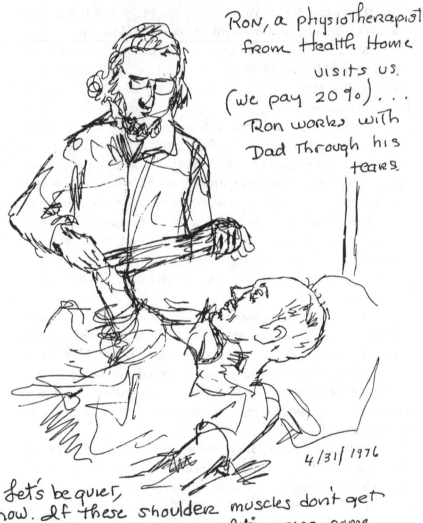

Ron, a physioTherapist
from Health Home
visits us.
(we pay 20%) . . .
Ron works with
Dad Through his
tears.

4/31/1976

"Let's be quiet,
now. If these shoulder muscles don't get
exercise They freeze up. It's gonna come
back but don't be in a hurry. Now Bob,
push the leg up and back." More tears
and "ooh-Ah-h's!"

OUR OWN PHYSIOTHERAPIST

April 31, 1976

Wow! Dad is better than we thought. Ron, our new physiotherapist, came this afternoon. He is short, slight, and aes-
thetic looking with wild black hair and a beard. He'll be coming three times a week.

Dad grumbled, growled, raised his eyebrows apprehen-
sively and shed some tears. When Ron sat him on the side
of the bed, Dad wanted to be transferred into the wheelchair
immediately.

"No. Let him sit up for awhile," Ron advised. "It's good for
him to sit up straight and learn to keep his balance without being in the chair. If he sits up more each day, and slowly moves
his torso in place for the next three weeks, he'll be able to sit
up longer each time when he is in the wheelchair, until he is
up more than he is down."

Ron demonstrated how to push Dad in a wheelchair going
down a ramp backwards and up a ramp forwards. "It's safer
this way, as the patient has less chance of falling out," he explained. He also showed us "range-of-motion" exercises, which
we are to do with Dad several times a day. Rose sat in on his
explanation and will be able to help out with the exercises.
Dad cried when Ron gave him hand exercises and circled his
fingers. "We must do more of this," Ron said. "There is little
pain, despite the tears, but the hand may hurt later."

Ron looked at the layout of Dad's room and told us that
the bed should be reversed. His paralyzed side should be away
from the door, so that all the action can take place on his good
side. That arrangement will make it easier to feed and bathe
him, and may make it easier for him to see us, as a stroke
patient's vision is often limited on the paralyzed side.

Ron said he doesn't believe a speech therapist is necessary at this time. Within three weeks his eye muscles will
be better and some speech may return on its own. (I learned
later that not all stroke experts agree.)

He showed us the best way to transfer Dad into a wheel-chair from the bed: "Have him place his good foot under the paralyzed leg while he is lying down; then he swivels the bad leg over the edge of the bed, using the good one. He presses down on the left elbow to lift himself up, and the aide then helps to swivel his body around and into a sitting position by placing her left arm under his legs and her right arm behind his shoulders or neck. The wheelchair is placed at an angle, right wheel towards the bed, and must be locked. When his legs are over the side of the bed, the aide should guide his shoulder so he is standing on his good leg. He then swivels, and sits."

Great! Now even Mother can learn to put him into a wheelchair. We must remember always to transfer Dad from his strong side. When we're returning him to bed, the chair must be placed at an angle so that the good left leg is closer to the bed. He stands, swivels and sits down on the bed.

RON'S DO'S AND DON'TS

1. Don't do everything for him.
2. Don't coddle him or use baby-talk.
3. Don't rush speech lessons immediately. Speech will come back according to his strength.
4. Do treat him like a man, even if he can't talk.
5. Do let him stand more to improve balance and strengthen his legs.
6. Do place a pillow under the heavy, paralyzed arm (which is in a sling), to relieve shoulder pain.
7. Do move the bed so action can take place on his good side. (Now he'll be able to make car transfers and eventually go to the beach which he loves).

Exercises for us to follow daily:

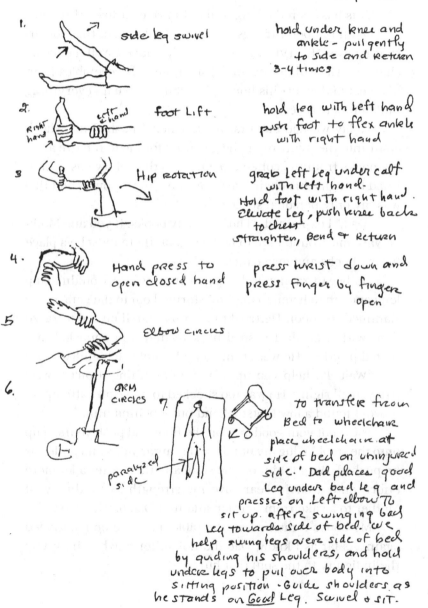

1. side leg swivel — hold under knee and ankle - pull gently to side and return 3-4 times

2. foot Lift — Right hand / Left hand — hold leg with Left hand push foot to flex ankle with right hand

3. Hip rotation — grab left leg under calf with Left hand. Hold foot with right hand. Elevate leg, push knee back to chest straighten, bend & Return

4. Hand press to open closed hand — press wrist down and press Finger by finger open

5. Elbow circles

6. Arm circles

7. to transfer from Bed to wheelchair place wheelchair at side of bed on uninjured side. Dad places good leg under bad leg and presses on Left elbow To sit up. after swinging bad leg towards side of bed. we help swing legs over side of bed by guiding his shoulders, and hold under legs to pull over body into sitting position. Guide shoulders as he stands on Good leg. Swivel & sit.

paralyzed side

FIRST FALL

May 1, 1976

This has been the longest day I have ever lived through.

Of all the petty things I hated in Dad, one of the most irritating was, "Everything must be ship-shape." Well, he hasn't changed. He still, for example, separates his vegetables from his meat and wants his home picked up as usual—everything in its proper place.

Today we had our first fight. When I pushed his wheelchair into the living room, he gestured for me to remove all of my books from the coffee table next to the yellow easy chair. I had brought this chair over from my Stuart house, and this was my only personal space.

"Dad," I explained. "Those are my books. If you and Mother want me around here to help you out, there must be a place for my books and magazines."

He began raving and I began fuming. He wouldn't stop long enough to listen to me, so I stormed out to the garage and slammed the door. He tried to get up and fell on the terrazzo floor with a crash. I rushed back to find him sprawled in a seated position. He was stunned and silent. I felt guilty.

"Wait. I'll help you up. Don't do anything. Don't worry! Are you all right?" He was too shocked to make any attempt to move. I found a low footstool and put it behind him.

"Now put your good arm on the floor and push yourself up onto the stool." I dug my hands under his armpits and pulled as he pushed. We got him on the stool and then, after a lot more effort, onto a chair. Fear gave me strength as I didn't want Mother to awake from her nap and find Dad on the floor.

My books remained on the table, never to be mentioned again. As far as I know, Dad did not suffer much pain. It was the indignity to the soul that hurt.

FRIENDS CAN HELP

May 9, 1976

Today, Mother and I came home from church to find a beautiful dinner on the sun porch. Friends have been kind. Some phone, others visit.

Several of Dad's friends, however, have found his stroke too difficult to face. Mr. Q. visited him in the hospital and went home ill from shock. Another gentleman, one of his best friends, just stopped visiting altogether. We later found out that he was a heart patient and feared a stroke himself. The poor man died of a heart attack a year later.

* * *

Don has come. This evening he is playing the piano and I feel I have found a family again. The deep sense of being unloved by my parents, even though I am taking care of them (or perhaps because I am), has abated for a moment. The hurt is being soothed and love is flowing in. Tears are flowing down my face as Don plays the same old songs Mom used to play: "Trees," "Claire de Lune," etc.—but with more zest. Both Mom's piano playing and singing are getting weaker. But she was the one who gave us three children an appreciation of music.

Bob used to play the violin. He is four years younger than I and I never considered him to be a threat. Don, however, could play the piano with an innate flair. He learned chords from our Swiss teacher as easily as he learned to swim.

I, on the other hand, had great difficulty understanding my piano teacher's accent and had to ask over and over exactly what she meant. I finally gave up in disgust and later learned to play by ear, but only in the key of "C." I used to sing while Mom played the piano and Bob played the violin. Dad sat by the piano, listening, as he is now. Twenty years later, I became a professional singer, performing from Greenland to South America in an act "Portraits in Song." I sketched a portrait while singing.

Dad is waving his good arm now and singing in time with

the music. Amazing! He can harmonize, even if he is not sing-ing the words. Mother stops playing and wants to put Dad to bed. Too bad! I don't see why he can't go to bed a bit later. I'm the one who has to get him ready for bed, anyhow.

Mom and I are having a battle of wills. She is fighting to be independent and to be the "boss," but she often has to lean on me. In the morning before the aide comes, Dad often screams and points wildly. If she doesn't understand him, Dad will sometimes grab her by the arm and turn her angrily in an attempt to make his wants clear. This only scares her. I often come to her aid and try to interpret what he's trying to communicate, which could be anything from "I want my face washed" to "The window should be opened wider."

At night, after the aide leaves, the same routine is repeat-ed, and as much as she tries to help, she only makes him more upset. Dad and Mother argue over how much to open the win-dow or whether he should have a blanket, as Mom insists, or simply a sheet, as he wants. I often agree with Dad, arguing that "He knows what he needs, Mom. Don't try to push him."

Don tells me I have done a good job, and it is good to be appreciated. We have all done a good job. But I often think of the twenty "Beatitudes" paintings I created four years ago. They almost foretold the anguish we have experienced with Dad's stroke. We have all lived "Blessed are they who mourn," as we walk in the valley of the shadow of death. We watched my father as he was crucified—and were crucified along with him.

Watching Oral Roberts, Sunday, May 10, 1971

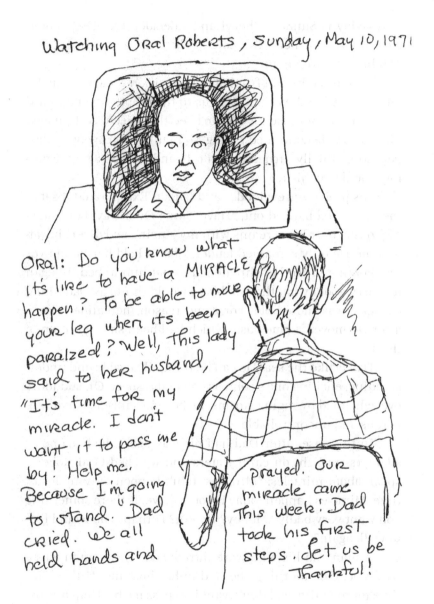

Oral: Do you know what it's like to have a MIRACLE happen? To be able to move your leg when its been paralzed? Well, this lady said to her husband, "It's time for my miracle. I don't want it to pass me by! Help me. Because I'm going to stand." Dad cried. We all held hands and prayed. Our miracle came this week! Dad took his first steps. Let us be Thankful!

LEGACY OF LOVE

May 10, 1976

Today is Sunday. Cheryl and I decided that Dad should look at the Oral Robert's Show. As he can't go to church, we will bring church to him.

We pushed him in front of the television set and turned it on. He raved and motioned for us to turn it off. I wondered if he was upset because he couldn't see the screen, so I pushed him closer. He continued raving, so I pulled him away. In desperation, I finally turned the set off—and then on again. Nothing would stop his raving!

His protests grew louder and wilder. Exasperated, I sat at the piano and banged out, "Have Thine Own Way, Lord," trying to ride over his screams with my singing and divert his attention. He only screamed louder. Cheryl held her hand over his mouth and Mother threatened to put him to bed. I began to worry about what the neighbors would think, as Dad's lung capacity was incredible. For some reason, he calmed down after we moved a blue vase, which had been sitting on top of the TV.

Dad is like the sea. He can be tranquil, lovable and understanding, eliciting one's compassion and respect. Or, suddenly overwhelmed by raging storms, he becomes irascible, cantankerous and uncontrollable.

In this case, after Dad had his way again, he became as silent as sunlight on calm waters and watched Oral Roberts speak about miracles: "Miracles didn't happen only in Jesus' time. Miracles happen today if you believe. Is there something you want very badly? Money? Health? Perhaps you would like to walk again?"

A man and his wife were introduced. The woman was a paralytic. One morning she said to her husband, "I think it's time for my miracle. I don't want it to pass me by. Help me, because my leg is going to move." She then stood up and walked. Mom, Cheryl, Dad and I wept together because this week Dad actually took his first few steps with Ron's help—thanks to Nelson, Cheryl, Annabel and God.

This was one of the few television programs we have watched in five years. Dad never liked TV and we seldom put it on. For this reason above all, seeing Oral Robert's show today about a paralytic is another miracle.

SPEECH THERAPY

May 11, 1976

Today a pert, cheerful blonde breezed in, bringing hope to all of us. Immaculate, every hair in place, she wore a crisp yellow dress and approached Dad with a winning smile.

"This is your speech teacher, Dad," I said. "Her name is Carol."

"How do you do, Mr. Thurston. Can you say your name?"

"Wa-wa," Dad rolled out the words, trying to comply.

"Bob," she enunciated carefully. "Watch my mouth."

"Wa," Dad uttered.

"Good. Now can you count from one to five? One, two, three, four, five."

"Ahh, Ooo, Eee ..."

"Good. You're saying vowels. We'll have to learn how to put consonants before them." She took out some play money and told Dad to give her one dollar. He picked it all up, and she put it down again.

"Give me $2." He gave her two.

"Give me $3." He gave her three.

"Very good." She took out several cards with pictures on them and laid them before him.

"Show me the butterfly." Dad pointed to the picture.

"Show me the hairbrush." He couldn't find it, nor could he pick out a dog. He could, however, point to the right colors she asked him to find. Dad had trouble understanding numbers, which is hard to believe because he has been "reading" the stock market page every morning.

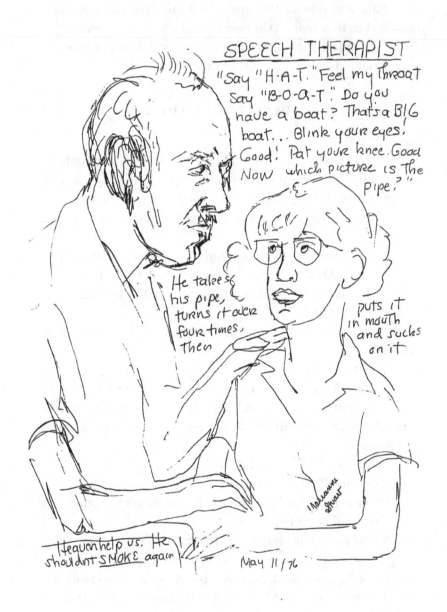

"His attention span goes in and out," Carol told us. "Stroke patients may hear only part of a sentence. It's best to speak to them with nouns first and then add the verbs. Don't use too many little words." How strange, I reflected, that he can't identify objects and pictures. Mom and I have been reading aloud every night and I wonder how much he has really understood. He seems to laugh and cry in the right places, but perhaps looking at a picture is different than creating a picture in your head of the spoken word. Speaking, listening, reading and writing are four separate tasks related to different parts of the brain.

"Look at my mouth. M-m-m-m-m. Make the sound." She put his fingers on her throat so he could feel the vibrations of an "M."

"Wa-wa!"

"Try 'ha.' Pop the air out." Dad blows.

"Almost. Let's try a sound that uses the tongue. Look at my mouth and watch the tongue rise." She spoke an "L" and then tried the "K" and hard "G" sounds. Dad tried to mimic her, but produced only more "Wa-wa" and "Eee-" sounds.

"Let's see if you can follow instructions," Carol said. "Blink your eyes." Dad does and Carol laughs. "I'd like you to pat your knee." He does.

Carol displayed some pictures. "Show me the pipe. You can smoke it." Dad points to a piano.

"You can't smoke a piano," she told him. "We're just trying to retrieve words," she explained to Mother and me.

"Now, point to the hat." Dad points to a boat.

I am depressed. My father, who has owned several boats in his life, cannot even recognize the picture of a boat. How can we, who have never had aphasia, possibly understand how devastating it is not to be able to speak—to say nothing of connecting words with objects.

Simple phrases such as: "I want a shave; turn off the light; I want the lawn mowed; someone's coming," can be communicated easily enough by pantomime or, in Dad's case, by roaring until we guess what he wants. But what of the more complicated emotions for which he has no words, such as: "I feel sad about my stroke. My life is over. I'm in a prison of despair. I resent every word you speak because I can say nothing. I resent also your anger, your frustration and your help."

Or perhaps he is thinking, "I am the father, the boss. Why does God take away my ability, my authority? It's my house! My bed! My body! My land! My wife!" .This was his attitude before the stroke. But now, perhaps, he is thinking: "It's not mine anymore. My home is run by strangers. People's faces are a blur from one to the other. Days melt into weeks and weeks slide into years. Only the growing grass is real to me—the sky, the river, the boats. Eating my dinner and spilling food on my bib is real to me. My daughter's anger and my wife's pity are real to me. But what is this monstrous thing that has happened to me, leaving me a poor excuse for a human being?"

A stroke, I conclude, happens not only to the stroke victim, but severely affects all of those around him. We suffer for and with the patient, feeling limited in our ability to communicate. Although Carol's presence today offers hope and help, it also brings a deeper sense of Dad's limitations.

"I can work with your father until he reaches a plateau," Carol explained before leaving. "I can keep coming as long as there is an improvement."

She left us a booklet, "Aphasia and the Family," from the American Heart Association, which includes the following passage: "The patient must be professionally assessed before speech therapy begins. The therapist must know the patient and his problem. Some aphasic patients may be unable to see or recognize pictures due to an excess of visual stimulus. Therefore charts may be frustrating."

She gave us essential rules for dealing with speech-damaged patients:

1. Never stop and talk unless you have time to listen.
2. Speak to the patient as you would speak to any normal, intelligent adult.
3. Speak slowly and do not raise your voice.
4. Never give pen and paper and ask him to write it if he can't.

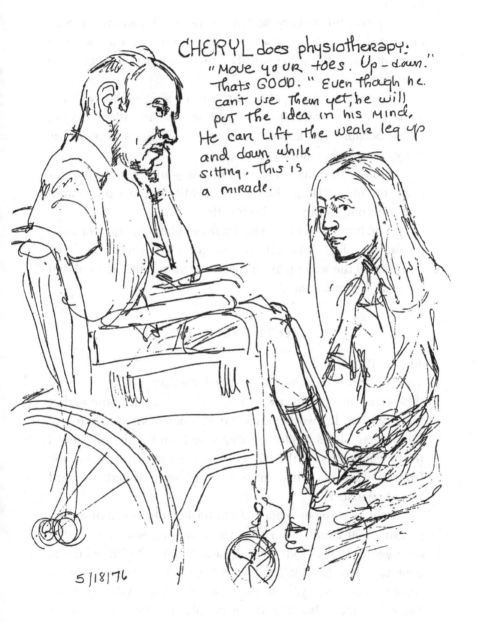

CHERYL does physiotherapy:
"Move your toes. Up - down."
Thats GOOD." Even though he
can't use them yet, he will
put the idea in his mind.
He can lift the weak leg up
and down while
sitting. This is
a miracle.

5/18/76

LESSON IN CONCENTRATION

May 18, 1976

Cheryl and Dad are seated on the porch together. I peek around the corner to observe. She is giving him a lesson in concentration. Kneeling calmly before him, she projects confidence and charm.

"Move your leg to the side, Mr. T," she intones. "At the same time, be aware of your hand on your leg. It's not going to fall because you know it is there." Dad begins to jiggle his body, revving his motor. He cries.

"S-h-h. Put your concentration on your leg, not your energy into tears." He pushes the leg gently with his good hand, and then moves the right leg a little.

"The hand won't fall. Don't worry." She puts the bad hand on the good leg. "Now lift up your good leg. It won't fall. Lift your leg all the way up but be aware of your hand. It won't fall because you are aware."

TO THE GARAGE

June 1, 1976

For three months I have been carting a heavy electric typewriter around in my van, so I can write at home and at Mom's. I live in two places at once. I never know where my underwear, shoes or clothes are. Now I am finally ensconced in the garage, using the old bed and bureau, which Don took from Dad's room when installing his hospital bed. A board serves as a desk.

I am working on a book about India, polishing stories and juggling 500 pages of writing and drawings which I created on my yoga tour of India with Swami Vishnu DeVenanda. The book is called "It's Not Too Far: A Yoga Tour of India." I took a six-week course in yoga at the Sivananda Yoga Ashram in Val Morin, Canada (1972), and am deeply indebted to India for her science of Hatha Yoga, which helped to rid me of arthritis pain, hyperventilating attacks and excess weight. Through breathing exercises, asana postures held steady, a vegetarian diet, and the art of relaxation, concentration and meditation, I attained improved health of mind, body and spirit.

Yet I had almost as much fear and ignorance about traveling to India as I had about my father's stroke. Both were walks into the unknown, for India was a far country to me, mysterious, frightening and different. Having a deep respect for its culture, I inwardly feared I might never return. Perhaps living in an ashram, studying and meditating, would bring me such joy that I would become a "Yogini." Instead, I returned to teach yoga in America. Teaching yoga, art and drama in my studio, my time is pretty much my own and I am free to help Mother when she needs me.

I've had several stormy scenes with Dad when he has seen the garage light on and screamed to have it put out. Tonight I exploded in anger.

"But I'm working out there, Dad. I need a place to live and work and that's where I'm working. I'm not going to turn the light out." He kept raving. We are so much alike that when our tempers mount, it is difficult for either of us to back off.

I remember one time when he upbraided me in our Maine cottage: "Take all your things upstairs," he ordered, "and don't let me see them downstairs again." How unfair, I had thought at the time, for my parents had a small room downstairs where they kept their clothes and we three children had to go upstairs for a change of shoes, a bathing suit, or a sweater. Some old button was pushed in my emotional facade and I screamed at the top of my lungs, "I didn't ask to be born!" This shocked and silenced them and Don had to play the peacemaker.

Now the same old resentment flared. I was fighting for my dignity, my self-respect and my survival. How could I remain here and help out in an impossible situation if I had no place to live? If only Dad had built a third bedroom or added the breezeway and a small apartment for family and visitors. Smart man! I guess he knew it would be difficult to oust family or friends who wanted free bed and board and a beautiful view of the Indian River.

But how can one argue with a damaged brain? Dad was single-minded before his stroke and now is even more so. Our voices rise harshly and neither will give in. I wonder if it's the old rational Papa speaking about wasting electricity, or is it that he hears the typewriter and is disturbed? We are at an impasse. I slam the door and return to my desk.

I shall try to make this my headquarters and, hopefully, will find time—and quiet—to write.

READING AND WRITING

June 2, 1976

Dad is learning to read and write again. We print our names in large letters and he painstakingly copies them with his left hand. He is right handed, so this is no small feat. Today I bought him a child's game called "Sesame Street Lottery Card Game." He seems to enjoy it as it is simple, colorful and fun. Part of an object is missing and he must identify it. The missing part is on the back of the card.

Dad has difficulty identifying words and objects. He is unable to point to the correct objects, so I wonder if he really understands when we read to him aloud. Often he has a dull, expressionless look which might mean confusion. But he makes us understand what he wants most of the time with persistence, charades and good old-fashioned hollering. He is so different from the Daddy I knew as a little girl—fastidious, silent, demanding, orderly, and time conscious. He can still tell time, but he can't count. Strange and wonderful—the complexity of the human mind.

We have been forgetting to give Dad the pills which the doctor prescribed to calm him down and thin his blood. I put notes on the refrigerator door and kitchen bar, hoping Mom will see them and remember pills when she brings in the food tray.

Dad's periods of raving are increasing. The doctor says the raving is the result of too little oxygen getting to his head. He explained that a cerebrovascular accident (CVA), can result in a clot in the artery or a rupture. In a cerebral embolism a piece of the clot breaks loose and plugs a blood vessel, causing paralysis of an arm and leg, lack of consciousness, or speech disorder resulting from a lack of oxygen in the blood. This may result in high blood pressure and hardening of the arteries. . . (I forgot to turn off the stove today, and sometimes forget letters to words when I'm writing. No doubt I should stand on my head more to bring blood and oxygen to my brain.)

I wonder if stroke patients go through the same phases of emotion that dying cancer patients do: denial, depression, anger, bargaining and acceptance. Dad's been through depression, now he's in anger. Will he ever get to acceptance?

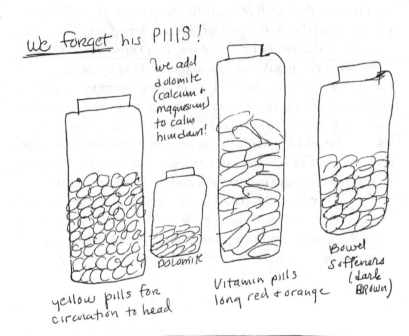

We forget his PIILS!

We add dolomite (calcium + magnesium) to calm him down!

DOLomite

yellow pills for circulation to head

Vitamin pills long red + orange

Bowel Softeners (dark BROWN)

We are FORgetting pills. He is having Raving times. Is it not enough oxygen to head? He drools, also. I put Notes on the Refrigerator door and kitchen Bar. Hopefully since Mom brings food in - she'll begin to remember!

Speaking of Memory ---- I forgot to turn off stove at My house today, after cooking a potatoe. Mom forgot I Had a potato and cooked another one for dinner - and I forget letters to wordsdim writing. I should, no doubt, stand on my head more!

DOMINOES

June 3, 1976

We play dominoes every night with Dad. Cheryl and the aides play with him in the daytime. It is one game he plays well, as he can read the dots and match them.

I tried checkers without much success since Dad will not follow the rules. He jumps backwards and forwards, and with great gulps of air and squeals of delight, confiscates his opponent's men. Although he seems to understand us, he is bull-headed enough to want to play the game his way, making up his own rules.

The worst problem, however, is our inability to understand him. When this happens, he gets superhumanly angry and I am grateful we live so far from the neighbors. They probably think we are harboring a caged wild animal, or, perhaps, even worse, think we are persecuting him. Sometimes Mother and I wonder if he might be better off in a nursing home. It certainly would be less tiring for us.

We are all in new roles. My karma is to be here—working two full days and being a backstop for Dad's anger mornings and evenings before the aide arrives and after she leaves. And at night, I am on call. Mother is Mother, friend, onlooker and decision-maker. Dad is child and boss-tyrant. Try as we may, we will never fully comprehend what is going on in that aphasic brain of his.

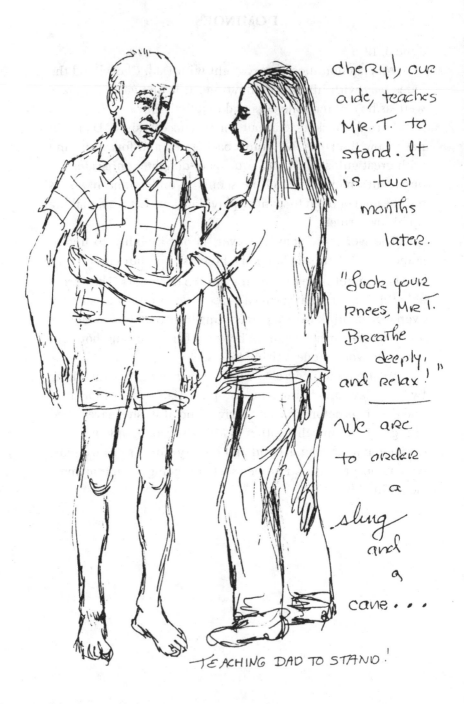

Cheryl, our aide, teaches Mr. T. to stand. It is two months later.

"Lock your knees, Mr T. Breathe deeply, and relax!"

We are to order a _sling_ and a cane...

TEACHING DAD TO STAND!

FIRST STEPS

June 4, 1976

And now for the good part. Dad is learning to walk at last! Today he actually took fourteen steps from his bed to the living room. Ron held on to the back of his pants and guided his shoulder as Dad, in his floppy slippers, painfully dragged his paralyzed leg through the hall and into the living room.

Never shall I forget the look of awe on his face. Tears streamed down his cheeks and his mouth hung open as he stared dumbly at his world. He took in the piano, his easy chair, the couch, dining room table, and the glistening river dotted with sailboats.

Dad was standing and walking for the first time. He was becoming whole. He was a survivor. Not a stroke victim, but a victor. His illness is a cross we have all had to bear. But now the miracle is beginning to happen. God is mending the body and the mind along with it.

I have been reading books on stroke, both for information and hope. Mother won't open the books. She has not faced reality enough to want to know the truth but prefers to live in a dream world, a world in which Dad will get totally "back to normal." It is, perhaps, this quality which will help her survive the ordeal of a stroke in the family.

BALANCING THE BOOKS

June 5, 1976

Dad's best friend, Ray Owens, came this afternoon to help Mom balance the books. As a child, I remember Dad hunched over his black mahogany desk trying to balance the budget. How often he screamed at Mother because she had no idea where the money went. Money management was not one of her talents.

"Polly, you can't think!" Dad's heavy voice shriveled us with fear. Mom would act apologetic, ignorant, and finally exasperated, as though Dad were at fault for even asking her to account for the money. The daughter of a doctor, Mother had lived in a twenty-three room house in Brookline, Massachusetts, with three maids and a butler and was surely never conscious of money or where it went. She never knew scarcity until the Depression when Dad was forced to borrow money from his father and took years to pay it back. He was frugal, exact and proud.

Mother may have cared little for balancing books or accounting for pennies (and even less for cooking), but she was generous with her love, kindness and attention, particularly where books, music, clothes, church and parties were concerned.

The word "money" has long put fear into my heart, for every time we three children heard our parent's voices raise in a fight over money, we hovered over the upstairs banister, sure that they would fight for the last time and split up. We thought they could not love each other if they yelled like that, and we would soon be out on the street, motherless and penniless.

Now the accounts were royally screwed up. But Ray's delightful personality made this seem unimportant. His radiant face and kind disposition were a healing balm to our troubled household. "Isn't it wonderful what a stroke can do for members of the family?" he purred happily, upon entering the living room. My eyebrows shot up as my brother Bob, who was visiting, answered:

"Yes. We were always afraid of my father before the stroke. He was dogmatic and demanding. Now the tower has toppled and our fear is gone. We are able to show him more love."

"The mountains shall be leveled and the valleys filled," I thought. These words sum up our lives. This stroke has brought mingled emotions—hope, fear, depression, anger, sorrow, and elation. We have been frustrated to the point of tears. Many times I have wished for peace and harmony, to be able to see through the glass—clearly. But tempers flare so rapidly that Mom and I lose sight of the invalid upon whose lives our emotions are hinged.

I am reading "Episode," by Eric Hodgins. He makes several important statements, which I have shared with Mother: "Responsibility for care must be shifted gradually to the patient. This is the essence of the problem psychologically. The brain is damaged. The patient experiences psychological regression, becoming childish and overly dependent. Slowly he will have to become a mature person again. You cannot hurry these things, according to the disability. His wife must be staunch enough to assume this responsibility in the beginning and willing to shed it later on as an essential feature of her husband's recovery. 'Oh, you poor darling,' is worse than useless! Make the patient comfortable."

What angers me is Mom's pity for Dad. If she could only accept his aphasia and paralysis as a part of him. Just ignore it, relating to the real Bob as she knew him, or the Bob he could become! Weeping only confuses the issue, and causes the problem and its anguish to persist. It keeps you stuck in your own self-pity.

WE HAVE a VISITOR. Oskar, I named him. Dad spotted him on the lawn. Shari brought him on the porch. He waddled and walked and pushed his way across the terrazo floor, jutting his head into The

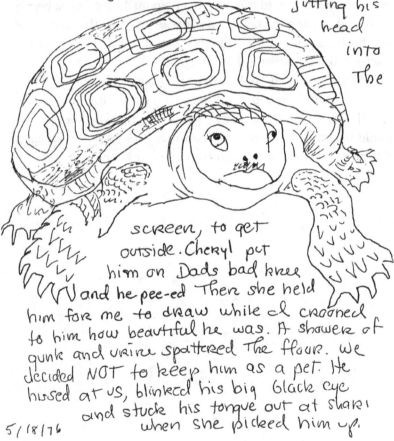

screen, to get outside. Cheryl put him on Dads bad knee and he pee-ed Then she held him for me to draw while I crooned to him how beautiful he was. A shower of gunk and urine spattered the floor. We decided NOT to keep him as a pet. He hissed at us, blinked his big black eye and stuck his tongue out at Shari when she picked him up.

5/18/76

OSKAR

June 6, 1976

We had a visitor today, a turtle I immediately named "Oskar." Dad spotted him on the lawn and Cheryl brought him up to the porch. He waddled across the terrazzo floor, butting his head against the screen in his attempt to get back outside. Cheryl placed him on Dad's bad knee and he peed. Then she held him for me to draw while I crooned how beautiful he was. A shower of gunk and urine spattered to the floor. He hissed at us, blinked his big black eyes and stuck out his tongue.

We decided not to keep him as a pet.

DON RETURNS

June 10, 1976

Don is here a second time. He is giving Dad a bath this morning, encouraging him to wash all of the parts he can reach. Dad buttons his shirt alone and puts on the sling. Letting him accomplish this takes more patience and time on the part of the aide, but it's valuable for a feeling of independence.

Watching Don with Dad, I realize that he has a great deal of compassion, as well as the ability to make Dad laugh. How I wish I had this easy rapport with Dad; I've always found it difficult to communicate with him. A friend told me that the child who stays home to care for the parent is often scorned because the parent resents the loss of power and his own child-like dependence. The siblings, however, are welcomed when they return. This certainly seems to be the case in our household.

Occasionally, however, Don's power of communication with Dad breaks down. This afternoon, for example, he tried to fix the power mower while Dad sat on the screen porch making gestures and uttering guttural sounds until it looked as if he might have an apoplectic fit. Don is hopeless with mechanical objects. "Is it this? Is it this?" he asked repeatedly, thinking it was good therapy to involve Dad, who only became increasingly frustrated. Luckily, my friend, Jerry appeared and fixed the machine.

We are trying to teach Dad the names of objects. I cut out color photographs and write the name under the object—e.g. baby, shirt, tree, children, boat, etc. It's difficult to know, however, if he is learning anything.

THE LOVE HALL

June 11, 1976

Tonight, Cheryl told Dad, "We're all going to church together. Those who pray together, stay together."

"But is he ready for an emotional experience like that?" Mother asked anxiously.

"God will take care of him," Cheryl answered.

Mother became rebellious. "Dad doesn't want to go," she said, meaning that she herself did not want to go and be embarrassed if Dad cried in public. Try as we might, we could not reason with Mother. Again it seemed a question of wills.

Cheryl was heartbroken and I was angry. I knew that this congregation had been praying for Dad all during his convalescence. What a miracle it would have been, and a victory for Cheryl, if Dad could have walked down the aisle to sit in the congregation.

Don, Cheryl and I went alone to the Pentecostal meeting at "The Love Hall." I am grateful for the prayers and support that the church members have been giving to Cheryl, for there has been love in our house, underneath all the pain.

There were only fifteen or twenty people seated in the converted garage. Don loved the singing, but thought there wasn't enough prayer.

Perhaps they were wary because the last time I had been there, I had let out a piercing shriek and then seemed to go into ecstasy. A smile was on my face and there was joy in my heart as I looked upwards into the light, my arms raised in praise. Everyone had then gone to the back of the church and proceeded to make the sign of the cross on my chest. Cheryl explained later that perhaps some people thought my scream meant that the devil was in me. The only devil I believe in is the devil of "ego" and negative thinking. People are strangely different.

LETTER TO AN AUNT

June 11, 1976

Dear Aunt Spud,

I am writing to you in confidence as I want an objective view of Mother before she breaks. I've been living with Mother and Dad, helping to care for both of them. It has been cumbersome, as there are only two bedrooms. Mom has the master bedroom and Dad is in the lavender guest room. I sleep in the garage or on the living room couch.

This has been a beautiful growing experience with Dad. He cries a lot and can't talk. He has outrageous tantrums, is depressive, etc. I've considered it all a blessing in disguise as he used to be so negative and harsh and now he is dependent. In a way it is helping Mother to gain an identity, or an independence which she never had before, although God knows that paying bills and balancing books has never been her strong point.

I feel closer to Dad, helping him bathe, dress, potty and walking him several times a week (it is a miracle that he is walking, with help), but I am having difficulty relating to Mother. She is often dictatorial and negative towards me. She holds so much resentment and pushes her "authority," not bending an inch to listen, seek or compromise.

For example, we argue over Dad's diet. She gives him all the salt and fats: butter, milk, eggs, meat and ice cream, every night. The books I have read on stroke warn us that this diet will lead to another stroke. Her response is always, "We did it this way all our lives and what's good enough for my parents is good enough for me." She believes that her way is the right way and the only way. Yet she suffers from high blood pressure and Dad has had a massive stroke.

Why is she so angry? Is she jealous because I am trying to run things? I am only trying to help. I feel like a blank piece of paper. I am here to help Dad walk, talk, communicate, to protect Mom from his anger, also to prevent her from overprotecting him. I can't see why she's so hateful and resentful.

Jesus! I never had a father until this illness. I can see him better now and the fear we children had of our father is lessened as we work with him. Our mast has toppled. Love is coming through from him to us and us to him. We are free to care and see truthfully, knowing he is a child of God. Mother always radiates in the presence of men. I know she was the prettiest of four girls and much loved by her family but was she always this insecure?

"I love my husband and always will," she declares. Funny, I always thought he was hurting her as we grew up, yet all the anger he displayed towards her has never made a dent in her outward show of affection. I admire her persistent, joyous optimism and her basic intention for him to get well. When we argue about diet I say, "He may be *your* husband but he's *my* father, and I do care about his health." We need Light, Light, Light!

Please tell me how you see your sister. I cannot see her clearly. Love and Light. Doris

ARGUMENTS

June 12, 1976

What a tinderbox! I went to my home in Stuart last night because I was so angry at Mom. I told her that she was selfish for not letting Dad go to church with us.

"You didn't come because you didn't want to. He was ready," I said venomously. "He loved it when I invited several young people in to sing religious songs one evening. They sang and clapped and prayed and Dad was thrilled. How can you keep your husband from his good—from people who have prayed for him?"

I was furious at her for not taking a step, and for "pulling her rank" on us, when Cheryl and I had helped Dad so much in his rehabilitation. Although things were calmer here today, there were still hurt feelings, anger, and frustration underneath. The poor patient is no longer the problem, but those around him, who are fighting each other over what they want to see done. Yes, this truly is the devil of the ego.

Tonight Mom took me aside and said, "I'm sick of your taking charge. You're just jealous of Bob, Don and Dad." I was shocked. Does she understand that I want her love? What child wouldn't want a mother's love? Why can't she give it to me? If I am jealous, who has made me so? Since she brought it up, could it be she who is jealous? It's all so confusing.

"We shouldn't fight, for Dad's sake," I pleaded. "We need harmony here or else I should go away. I've only tried to help, but you take offense at everything I do." I followed Mom to her room and she hit me on the back and closed the door. I followed her in.

"I'm *not* jealous of you," I seethed. "I never wanted to be in your shoes when I saw the way Dad treated you. I never wanted marriage or a husband. I didn't want to be a servant, a slave to someone else's whims."

"But Doris, he is my husband. I've loved him all these years and I'll always love him." Could she mean that? What strange shapes love takes. How wrongly I interpreted her feelings. She meant, of course, "I'll stick by him even if it kills me." And it damn well may!

"But mother, he's my father. Here's what we're arguing over ... possession, power. Yoga says it's "I-ness and my-ness" that causes all the problems, conflicts and pain in life. He isn't mine or yours, he's God's."

"Oh, I'm sick of your preaching," she answered caustical-
ly. "Don't preach to me."

There is no communication here, no sharing. Why do we
fight over a wounded man, a changed, helpless human being
with whom we all have trouble communicating? What is there
so commanding about Dad's personality that makes us want
to help him to the exclusion of everyone else? How soon before we all will ignore him and wait for the other to help?

My insides are churning with anger. I must go home again
tonight and leave Don in charge. Today Don told Cheryl how
sweet Dad is. Unbelievable! So the softness is coming through
to him, too. We are all rediscovering our Pop, despite the jealousy between Mother and me, and possibly Don.

"WA-WA'S" OF HAPPINESS

June 13, 1976

Cheryl has gone and I will miss her. She told Mother she
wanted a raise but Mother wouldn't agree. I think, personally,
that Cheryl has done her job and there is no more challenge
here. Dad is walking and the days have become tedious, so she
is moving on.

We have a new aide. Pearl, a glowing black woman with a
cheery disposition and merry smile comes well recommended. Her spirit has mellowed us all. She acts as housekeeper,
aide and cook, but can come only twice a week.

Today she walked Dad all around the house, holding on
to the back of his pants. Don walked alongside Dad, who in-
dicated that he wanted the bushes trimmed by slicing his left
hand horizontally and snipping with his fingers. When Dad
saw the hedges trimmed and the backyard mowed, he raised
his head and bellowed with pleasure.

Don is finding a father. He does a good job of bathing Dad
and uses quiet, slow, simple phrases with humor when exercising him.

DON IS LEAVING

June 17, 1976

I drove Don to the airport in Palm Beach for his flight to New York. As he stretched out his hand to say goodbye, my heart wrenched in despair. He had been here for ten days, ten days which diminished me. Perhaps I have always been diminished by this radiant, sunny, ebullient soul—part man, part pixie, part brother, part God.

In helping us care for Dad, he filled up the crevices of doubt, suspicion, loneliness and misunderstanding, shedding light, joy and empathy along with his stern reprimands. He brought hope and love. His buoyant humor and gentle spirit contain a profound respect for life.

After watching Cheryl bathe Dad, he gradually took over, becoming an excellent male nurse. "I love it," he said. "I would have liked to become a male nurse if I weren't already a political science teacher."

Watching him walk away, tall, erect, handsome and newly tanned, I remembered the little baby brother I used to shelter and protect in Houston. Now he was looking after me. My little brother of the quick dimples and laughing lake-blue eyes was growing up. His ruddy face, imprinted with lines of living, feeling and loving, was in contrast to that of his older brother, Bob. Like the Virgo that he is, Bob's round, moon face is handsome in a different way, untouched by life and virginal, containing all his emotion within the fortress of his body.

Looking back ten days ago, I recall the first moment when Don appeared in our kitchen doorway, bag in hand. Helpless and apprehensive, he did not know what to expect or how he would respond. He had inquired of his friends about stroke patients, but nothing could prepare him for the reality he must face alone. A father he had known as dominant and tyrannical, whom he couldn't get close to, was now partially paralyzed and unable to talk.

This might be his last chance to communicate with a man

he barely knew, a man at whose side he had often worked in silence, a man who was exacting, cryptic and impatient, a father whose constant demands for perfection often lessened our belief in ourselves.

There was no need for words when Don played the piano. Running through Dad's favorite composers—Bach, Beethoven, Liszt, Chopin and Schubert—he played with strong, measured exuberance, filling the house with emotion and beauty as if nothing had changed. Dad sat at his side in the easy chair, head down, entranced.

In addition to becoming adept at caring for Dad, Don also added his pithy comments in the evening over a game of checkers or dominoes, matching Dad's victorious yelps with roars of laughter. He communicated for long periods of time in silence, seated on the porch or on the lawn watching the sailboats go by, and verbalizing dramatically when necessary, enunciating clearly when he failed to interpret Dad's finger gestures. Laughter followed.

Although diminished by his presence, I am also completed. It will be difficult to fill the void left by my younger brother.

"WOW-WOW'S" OF DEPRESSION

June 18, 1976

Dad went into a glum, hopeless shell after Don left, responding neither to Mother nor me. A stony resentful silence lay between us at the dinner table. Perhaps it *would* have been better if Don had never come, as the cure seems worse than the problem.

I feel my presence irritates Dad. All through the evening meal he is silent, neither smiling nor lifting his head. Mom is "very-gooding" Dad. She is learning to praise him, which is what Don told us we needed to do. Don also explained that Mom and I fight each other because we do not appreciate one another.

I have to keep reminding myself that underneath all the

terror, hostility, frustration and bruised egos, there is only love. After dinner, Dad wailed when I played "Claire de Lune," and cried bitterly when Mom tried to read to him. His protestations seemed louder than usual and irritated me, perhaps because we two women can find no way to meet his needs.

I gave him a simple cutout puzzle but he waved it away as being childish. Yet, at the same time he pointed out two places where the pieces fit. I haven't taken care of him now for two weeks and feel unable to communicate.

The house is haunted by Don's sweetness. Our loneliness rattles around in a joyless space. All I can offer is tears and anger.

Mother is putting him to bed and he is "wow-wow-wow-ing" about his pills, followed by a loud guttural "ah-ah." Next it will be the windows. She does not give him enough air and I'll have to go in and fight for him to have a few more inches, which Mom will say causes too much of a draft.

REHABILITATION CENTER

June 19, 1976

I visited the Rehabilitation Center for Crippled Children and Adults in Palm Beach. If I had my way, I would take Dad immediately for evaluation and possible therapy, hopefully Occupational Therapy. In "Activities for Daily Living" he would learn to dress himself, go to the bathroom alone, shave himself, etc. The Rehabilitation Center has a swimming pool for physiotherapy. Water therapy is a valuable motivator and adjunct to physical therapy.

Dad could go with the consent of his doctor. Home Health would not object as long as the Center offers therapy that Home Health doesn't offer. Bicycles, weights, hot packs, parallel bars are included in a written schedule for daily therapy drawn up for each patient after an evaluation.

Mother vetoed the idea because she thinks it's too far for Dad to go. Yet she is considering taking him to Maine!

LETTERS OUT

July 20, 1976

Dear Brothers:

I am trying to untie the umbilical cord. I cry a lot. I visit the folks and get angry and leave. I guess I feel guilty. It takes ten years to grow from baby to teenager and another ten on the other end to be willing to accept old age and death.

I liked my new freedom after we got a new aide. Cheryl left us as she threatened to, and we hired two aides to alternate mornings. Also, a speech therapist comes twice a week from Home Health. Dad has become quite maniacal and his raving is a constant source of irritation. After he pulled Cheryl's hair, I believe she was a little afraid of him. So she has gone. Mission accomplished.

Dad won't let me do much for him. I can't read to him, help him get up, turn on the hose, or talk to Mother about bills. I have been a lowly dishwasher, cook, mail-getter, and assistant walker. I did therapy twice after Mom gave him a tranquilizer. Sometimes I think he should take this pill for a week as he cries and shouts so much. This constant "Wa-wa-wa" gets on my nerves and drains me emotionally.

Mom tried to tell me this, but not until I moved in was I able to understand. Now she has full care for two weeks and it's great she can do it and feel needed. She still treats Dad like a baby and continually tries to please him. I wish we had a strong man here to do therapy and shut him up.

I may go to Maine this summer along with you, Don, as it looks like Mom and Dad aren't going to make it this year. When I ask him if he wants to go, he shakes his head sadly, "No." (Mother is trying to do too much alone and Don and I agree, Bob, that if we both go to Maine, she may come to her senses and get full-time help again).

Love, Doris

August 15, 1976
Dear boys:

I'm driving north alone. Just called Mother from South Carolina and she has put Dad in the hospital. Maybe if he goes to a Convalescent Home afterwards, she can get a much-needed rest. Hopefully, she will then realize that she needs part-time or full-time help. Perhaps she can get Home Health again. Who knows, maybe when he returns he won't be so demanding.

I walked Dad before I left home and he kept getting his foot caught under tables and chairs, and not noticing. (I read that stroke patients with eye problems on the paralyzed side may bump into furniture they don't see). I suppose if he becomes too self- sufficient, Mother would worry about where he was and be afraid he would fall. I have tried to add pillows to elevate his chair so he can get up alone without help, but he will have none of it. The pillows get slung across the room.

Mom walks behind him holding his trousers and trying to curtail the distance. I think he has rejected therapy partly because she babies him so, yet you almost have to let him have his way because he is so adamant and vocal. I admire Mother's strength, however, and her determination. Dad bitched at her all her life and cut her down, and now she must be his strength and tower.

I've cried a lot—at my inadequacy, at Dad's. At Mom's getting stuck with him as an invalid. At watching them both go down so beautifully.

Love, Doris

August 19, 1976
Dear Brothers:

En route to Maine I stopped at Baba Muktananda's Ashram in New York and put down $200 towards a trip to India. I want to visit his ashram in Ganeshapuri, outside Bombay. Mom has been telling me to get out of the house. "Go, we don't need you here!" So I shall go if I can, although I don't really see how she can get along without me.

I drove north to recuperate at the Sivananda Ashram in Val Morin, Canada, where we practice yoga outdoors four hours a day with a glorious view of the Laurentian Mountains. When I sit in meditation I feel the power of Christ and the love of God flow through me, experiencing such ecstasy and bliss.

I feel close to the Eastern religions and think that Jesus studied with the Indian saints and sages. After all, "I am that I am," which is God's definition of himself, is in the early Sanskrit Teachings. I believe there is only One God and he created and loves us all, regardless of race, color or creed.

Love, Doris.

MY VACATION

August 24, 1976
Dear Folks:

I arrived at Norvega in South Brooksville, Maine one day before Don is to drive south to be with you. Please survive, Mom, for one more week. It must be tough caring for Dad alone. I really think you need a full-time live-in helper, and someone to eat with and talk to.

I have taken the downstairs room in the cottage and expect any moment to hear your voices: "Don't put that there ... Please get the wood ... Start the fire ... Sweep the floor ... Move your car ... Do the shopping."

My writing is spread out on the dining room table, as usual. The sun is a teeming red force in a tranquil, hazy sky. I think of Grandpa and Aunt Gwen, (those who have passed on), and the joy they felt sitting on the rocks overlooking Penobscot Bay and the thirteen islands.

Working with you and Dad, Mom, I have felt your interests narrow like a fading light. I have experienced the beauty of God folding the blanket after the peak of life. As one changes colors like a brilliant autumn leaf, fading in hue, so does the body return back to the elements from which it came—earth, water, fire, air and ether. But the soul remains strong and unchangeable, escaping the body only to come back again to continue its evolution towards God and Self-realization. Nothing in this life can disappear, only change form. We have within us all of the elements in this world. So truly our elements just change form . . .

I miss my cat. The flag pole is creaking; the wind chimes through the front door; the ocean is lapping, and the wood fire burns lustily. The Maine house is a treasure, and this place a legacy of beauty. The smell of pine, the rocks and the bay, the vibrant gray stillness of dawn on a placid sea, night stars and the Milky Way, and the terrible stately aloneness! Just being with nature. The rise and fall of morning and evening. No phones. No electricity. And kerosene lamps.

I feel Dad's presence in the rocking chair and you are here with me now, sitting on the porch staring into the blue bay. Watching the sail boat races, and the sky coming down -- majestic moving cinema of color. All the beauty of life is deep within us. We have only to shut our eyes and seek the ecstasy and Oneness within.

Dad, I know it is difficult for you to live in the prison imposed upon you but you have your eyes and your ears and you have love. That is the most important. For God never sends us burdens we cannot bear, or challenges we cannot meet, or crosses we cannot carry--with his help. I had to go away to get strong.

Life is exciting again.

Love, for now. Doris

P.S. Mother, if you really need me I can cancel my trip to India.

PART THREE

F<small>AMILY</small> C<small>OLLAPSE</small>

(October 1, 1976—August 29, 1977)

III

October 1976

THE STROKE

Strange to return to what I once called home
A broken man, my father—and alone
Encased in what was once a healthy frame
He now in livid anger cries and moans.

No more the power of word to grasp or use
No more to dim another's glowing fuse
No more the man, intelligent and proud,
The fruitful father becomes child ... abused.

What curse upon this body, noble head
Has thus benumbed his speech and heart, so dead?
Into what blackness, prison of despair
Has he been cast, to sudden torture wed?

This hallowed puppet, paralyzed with shame

No more to write, or spell or speak his name

Has thrust upon our lives a gloom of doubt

Encrusted with death's terror, power to maim.

And crippled as he is, we too become

Our body shocked with tears that flow, succumb

To half the person that we really are

And like his crutch, we live—and move, but dumb.

And dumb the child within us screams at God

Our anger fed by sparks from Father's rod

Who sheds us as God sheds his waning son

That soon may burst a new pea from the pod.

'Tis August, and the heat of summer's noon

Sends jeweled sweat and tears as added boon.

Pity, pain's accompanying blessed mate

Is prodding hearts, which Job has come to prune.

October 2, 1976

Mother wrote me to come home and I guess she needed me, after all. I cancelled my trip to India.

PROSTATE OPERATION

October 2, 1976

Dad has gone to the hospital for a prostate operation. I believe he is dying. The most excruciating part is that he cannot tell us about it. He is paper-thin. Was Jesus this way? There is nothing but the bones. He is being given intravenous feedings with tubes attached to his arms and legs. He has a catheter in his penis. His lips are blue; he chokes when he swallows. They give him oxygen twice a day.

OH, JESUS, HE'S DYING

Oh Jesus,

            he's dying

     he's dying

        and he can't

  talk.

He can't even

         tell

     us about it.

He's so thin.

    Jesus

      Jesus

        Jesus

Is this the way you were?

I didn't know

Oh, Christ

I didn't know

Nothing but the bones,

Lord

Nothing but the bones.

The doctor is happy

"Operation successful"

But the urine is so yellow . . .

"Incontinent."

October 3, 1976

He is still with us. Will he die here? God, do you cast this burden upon us because we are strong and you know we can take it? Or are you teaching us a lesson?

THE CLOCK STOPS

October 4, 1976

The living room clock has stopped. Mother never remembers to wind it, as that weekly chore used to be Dad's. The old mahogany clock has been a faithful friend, serving our family well for as long as I can remember—keeping time, organizing our lives. In some ways, Dad is now like that clock. Sometimes we wind him up too tightly and he shuts down. Other times he needs to be wound up or he will just sit. He needs more friends, more things to do. But where is the key?

As I place the clock's long gold key in the slot, I think of the events and occasions the clock has marked. I can hear my father calling us to come down to breakfast. It's time to go to school, time to play, time to meet Dad's train, time for the evening meal, time to do homework and time to go to bed. Deadlines. Order and togetherness out of chaos.

The clock begins chiming: two/one, two/two, two/three. The timing is off. Finally I set her small hands on eight and she slides into the right chiming. Ah, victory!

I wish it were this easy to bring Dad back to health again.

October 5, 1976

RAIN DIRGE

What makes the clouds so low tonight,

                dark rain

Culminating far too soon at twilight

Beneath the glowing rays of dusk

                the lightning

brief glimmer—shining bright

                amidst the gray.

Dark drifts of sky come down

Distant call of evening trumpet

Moon-haunted mountains edged

                with light

Your face—taut broken strings

                grimace

hedging on hospital pillow

Small trophies these, to

> still stay clean
>
> while eating

Raw, quick surge of tears

at what was once

> a man.

THREE PORTRAITS

My Father

He lies there, helpless beneath the rose-patterned blanket. Mouth open, the limp lower lip forms a wider gap on the paralyzed side of his body. An overgrown white mustache sprawls above the rim of the upper lip like weeds in an unkempt garden, changing the trim, dapper look of the country gentleman into the comfortable sweetness of an absent-minded professor. Now a grandfather, he wears the quaint demeanor of an unsure child. You approach him. The blankness begins. Stroke the balding head, feel the crisp sprigs of waning silver in the autumn of his life

"Hi! How've you been?" No response. Your words slide into a slower tempo. "Mother was here this afternoon, wasn't she?" The blank look—empty eyes.

"You know me, don't you, Daddy?" He is still staring. The head moves almost imperceptibly from side to side. "I'm your daughter—Doris." Tears, as the long face crinkles in frustration.

"Of course you know me. You just got mixed up about 'yes' and 'no,' that's all." Rub the paralyzed shoulder, press the thin arm. Take the unused hand, unused now for days, weeks, months. Try to bend the curved, stiffened fingers. His other arm responds weakly. The minute gesture, like the head nod, could be interpreted: "Don't work with my hand. Please take your arm away. Leave me alone."

"OK. But your arm needs a little circulation. Was the aide here today? Remember how she used to do this for you?" Place the crippled arm, so like a wounded animal, back in its cradle of sheets and blankets. He has responded, however dimly. He has not left you yet. One more attempt at communication. You hear his stomach gurgle. Thinness of a deteriorating old man. Now ask him to suck the juice with the straw. One more time. He blows it out on the roses.

"You're playing games. You blew it. Now suck it in—up. Try again."

Portrait of a man ... dying

Mother

A little woman in her late seventies...white hair framing the piquant, squarish face. Peaked eyebrows perch above piercing blue eyes. A small bird impetuously efficient at her project of the moment—her attention span momentary and fleeting. The body stoops a bit as she rounds the curve of middle age.

Now the forgetful woman, she is soon to become the child, caught in the transition from authority to helplessness. The bird can still sing, the face smile with the brilliance of the morning sun. A cheery disposition, except when daily anxieties and cares frazzle her edges like a frayed shawl. The knife of her tongue dulled to another's needs, she frets over immediate concerns, shutting you out again. Darkness.

Her mind has gone inward, chasing the rainbow of her own thoughts, leaving you able to enter your own private shrine, a world so different from hers.

Me

I am a "chip off the old block." Sad, angry, vengeful—with dark-brown eyes like my father's that dig into your soul. Some people are drawn into their warmth; others shy away from their sharp analysis.

An artist, I have communicated through painting, dance, poetry and song. I have sought to do that which pleases me. Mother may label me "selfish," my friends "talented," yet others—"crazy."

I am my father, my mother, and me. I am their conflicts, their love, their hopes, their despair and their anger. I am the bird flying into the unknown or the cat stalking out its territory. My life seems to be a search for space, free space—and love. I guess all three of us have been seeking love. And here we sit, impaired by each other. Fighting with each other and struggling with ourselves not to hurt each other.

Dad, of course, has an excuse.

THE RUBY RING

October 6, 1976

Today is my birthday and Mother gave me a ruby ring. I had begged her to let me wear my grandmother's diamond ring. Mom wears it now and then, but most of the time it's in her jewelry box.

My grandmother was very spiritually aware, very God-conscious, and I want to feel her protecting love and power. I need some support to get through these difficult days and feel that the ring would help. But Mother says no—I may wear it after she goes. How does she know she will die first? I need the harmony, strength and love now.

I recall the vision I had when I was forty-four. A Unity minister warned me that something tremendous and frightening would happen to me and asked if I were prepared.

"Yes," I replied. "I have been studying Jesus' teachings

and have been painting a series of dramatic oils based on the Beatitudes (Matthew V, vs. 1-9), interpreting scripture through word, color and movement."

All my life I had known God as energy. I had not been close to Jesus the man until I came to know him through dance and art. While choreographing dances to "Twelve Spirituals on the Life of Christ" for a motion choir of young adults, I performed the roles of Jesus and Mary and fell in love with Jesus. I realized that he had experienced every emotion known to man--sorrow, love, hate, anger, pride and joy. He had been there before me and was with me now. Yet I was unprepared for the majestic, terrifying vision of Christ enthroned, which came to me early the next morning.

Awakening at dawn, I noticed the cat was no longer sleeping at my feet, but was hunched up on my shoulder, hair bristling in fear. I saw nothing but a black ball. Three small balls of white light kept circling and expanding within it until they merged into a huge vision of Christ, enthroned. The image was three stories high and I, a speck of dust before him. He wore a crown on his head, and his eyes were beaming light. I was overwhelmed, and melted in His love. I saw no pupils and later realized He must have been meditating.

His arm reached out to me and, although there was no sound, I was aware that he was saying: "Don't worry." In Bible language this could be interpreted, "Peace, be still and know that I am God." I closed my eyes. When I opened them the vision was slowly fading and melting downwards as if someone were turning off a television set.

Too stunned to move, I finally touched the table beside my bed and realized that I had been given a new awareness. I knew now that what I could see, touch and hear was not real, but Life and Death were all one—a blue fire of energy. That is all.

Stumbling into my kitchen I looked through a window into my studio and was shocked to find a drawing of Jesus propped up against some books. I had drawn this twenty years ago at

Star Island, New Hampshire, after a meditation. Glen Clark, founder of Camps Farthest Out, and director of our religious conference, first taught me how to pray. Unbelievable!

Where had the drawing come from? Who placed it there? And why had the vision come to me? This was the same person I had seen in my vision. My inscription read: "Through word, pictures and movement, you shall bring people to me."

In the years that followed I began to paint my dances and dance my paintings. After sketching The Beatitudes from dances, I decided to interpret the drawings in color moods and painted twenty large, expressionistic oils.

As for the diamond ring, an aide must have stolen it, for it disappeared from Mother's jewelry box.

OCT 7, 5;30 AM

A little Lizard is on the screen outside my window in Stuart. I've had a week's vacation while "Bob" was in the hospital with prostate "digging" operation. Mom went every day for hours. She is being HONED to a tauter, firmer wire--- like a violin.

Looking at the LIZARD, I recognize the same LIFE-POWER in him... strong body of my.. hospital bed. the urge powerful. The surge of bodies Blends with the Live because this is the are driving at present-

as in The frail-father in his to Live is energy in our desire to vehicle we our BODY.

The day is waking and the earth is turning!

HOME AGAIN

October 7, 1976

Dad came home from the hospital, slower and weaker. Flesh hangs below his pasty buttocks and the bones stand out in his knees. It is hard to believe that illness can ravage a body in so short a time. Truly God is pruning us.

Dad seems drugged, but perhaps that's only because he is not uttering his usual loud "Ha-ha's." I just put a diaper on him and he didn't protest, but surprised me by helping to pull them up. I do not know this new father, this docile bed patient.

Dad, will you now become only a body? Your non-violence and cooperative muteness makes me dumb, also. I can't help but think that the best way out would be down. The nurse said you cried today and were sad because you've lost so much strength. You are like a dazed and wounded animal. We can only help you to die gracefully.

I am angry at Mother because she took away the night light and emptied the urine bottle. Now I can't see the color and quality so I don't know if I should give you water pills.

I quit, Dad.

I'm tired of being at your mercy. I'm ready for you to go and can see how easy your passing could be. Or will you transform unexpectedly back into the raging tiger? From sleep, will you surprise us again and leap back into health?

October 8, 1976

OUR CAPTAIN

My father was a handsome man, his ship

Was Clipper-tight, the hatches battened down

With care, the tiller held with might. No slip

When he was at the helm, our galleys bound

With fright. We listened to his orders brusque

And hastened, humbly bowing before him,

Authority unquestioned. Angry gusts

Of temper swept the breasts of kith and kin.

Feared, unbending, domineering power

Our rock, our guide, our goal—pinpoint of light,

And grateful, we leaned upon our tower

Assured and knowing he would win the fight.

Ship is sinking, tiller gone, rudder shored.

The mast has broken. Have we lost our Lord?

BREAKTHROUGH

October 9, 1976

Dad is skeleton-thin. I think he is dying. Standing by his bedside tonight, I gazed at the Lincolnesque bone structure, the sunken cheeks and watery, glazed eyes.

"Jesus, if he is dying I must talk to him and give him a chance to communicate his fear," I thought. How dreadful to be dying and to be unable to speak to another human being.

"Dad," I began, summoning all my courage, "Are you afraid?"

The nod was barely perceptible. I leaned closer to the still, silent form.

"Are you afraid of dying?" He nodded more emphatically and looked gratefully up at me in sudden acknowledgment. Thrilled at his response, I plunged on. "I know how you feel! I mean, I've been there!"

How could I tell him that only this morning while sitting in a dentist chair, I had been so consumed with the fear of his dying that I had hyperventilated. Struggling for breath, I felt as though I myself might die. The police came and refused to let me rest in my van, but insisted instead on taking me to a mental hospital. I was freezing and unable to talk or breathe. An irritating man in a white coat kept questioning me until I managed a choked scream:

"Get ... him ... out of here!" The hospital personnel later apologized to me for the ignorant way in which I'd been handled. Mom picked me up and although I tried to explain to her the stark terror that had consumed me and brought on the hyperventilation, she seemed only irritated. How strange, even with the ability to talk, I still couldn't communicate.

"Dad, I've been unable to breathe more than once," I said aloud. "And it's frightening. But it's going to be OK. Whatever happens, Dad, we will be with you. And we know what you are feeling."

Overjoyed, I ran into the living room to tell Mom what had happened. I had cut through the darkness of Dad's despair and allowed him to communicate his fear of dying to me.

"Mother, Mother! Dad's afraid he's going to die and I actually had a conversation with him. It's wonderful!"

She looked up, shocked, her blue eyes blazing in anger. "What do you mean, die?" she exploded. "Of course he's not going to die. Why should you tell him a thing like that?" She stormed into Dad's room on a rescue mission. I felt deflated. She had misunderstood me again.

"Bob, Bob!" She shook his paralyzed shoulder. "You're not going to die! Why, you're getting better every day. You'll be walking again in a few weeks and we're going to take you to Maine this summer. We'll be sailing again. You'll see."

I crept sheepishly back into his room in time to catch his slow vacuous grin. Although the incident had backfired, it helped clear the air and hope was born.

MY LIFE CLOSED TWICE

My life closed twice before its end
Kings and fountains little men
And deep within me one huge tear
Silent, unshed, was my gear

The river narrowed—life gave way
Her accomplice held at bay
The two together, holding hands
Lovers, moved at my command

Substance and shadow, life and death
Sun and moon of grief bereft
Sky and earth together clinging
Sorrow, webbed with laughter, ringing

Arraigned in momentary gleam
Incidents of life the theme
Towards one channel, depth meeting height
Love, hate, joy, pain, joined in flight

And now in poverty of peace
Action is stilled, and Being ceased.

NEW AIDE

October 11, 1976

Janice returned to work today. A slight brunette, she is half Dad's size. She has been very dependable, even though she loves her coke and cigarettes. We found her after putting an ad in the Stuart News for a "Housekeeper-Aide, stroke-aphasic patient. Experienced. Own transportation."

Several people phoned and I questioned them about their background, experience, age and hours available. Janice sounded the most amiable, so I invited her to our home for an interview and hired her.

It's amazing how she handles Dad. She is jolly and firm, and Dad likes her. She has done a good job exercising and walking him, but sometimes she appears sad and lifeless, upset at his setback.

IN THE BALANCE

October 12, 1976

Janice is here again today. She lifted Dad like a baby from wheelchair to bed and back again. The catheter is out. Dad is better, but must be turned every few hours. We are force-feeding him. He is aware enough to want to read the newspaper in the morning, but he can only read the numbers and turns immediately to the stock market reports.

Dad has been going steadily downhill for the past several months. He has passed through at least four of the phases of serious illness and death reported by Elizabeth Kubler Ross (disbelief, denial, depression and anger). We hope that when it's necessary, he'll move to the final phase—acceptance.

He has regressed to the point that a slight whimper is the only way he can express most of his needs. His head is slumped forward, perhaps indicating a return to his depression. He sleeps, is bathed, eats, goes to the bathroom, and eats and sleeps again. These are the final necessities of life. As we come into this world, so do we leave it-- with few needs. The clock is winding down. Our lives may be temporarily re-wound, our bodies momentarily aided by injections, feedings or pills, and we can be revived with oxygen. But sooner or later we must go.

Clock, who will be the first to give up? Time passes. I have tended you faithfully and you have kept order in our lives. But I have shrunk from the reality of time—for I wanted the timeless. I wanted to capture time by painting the essence of life, by painting eternity. Now as I grow older, I want *order*. All I have left are words. Into the abyss of time, these too will pass.

MOTHER IS ILL

November 3, 1976

I am sick to my stomach and sick in my heart. I will have a heart attack from anger at my parents. Why? Dad is better. He walks around the house and points to things to fix. But Mother is turning into a scarecrow with scrawny legs, her face cross-hatched with worry. Dad is often nasty and abrupt with her.

Mother had a numb arm and cheek this week and kept muttering, "Oh, my God. I'm going to have a stroke!" Janice rubbed her arm and face and kept telling her to relax, although she, too, was frightened.

I get angry at Mother because she tries to do everything. When I am getting a meal she is underfoot, trying to guide, question and suggest. She's driving me wacky and I have no patience with her. Perhaps she is at the end of her rope and I shouldn't be so nasty. I want her to rest more. How can one get through to her?

"Mother," I began this noon. "We could be friends."

"I thought we were," she retorted.

"Well, you disparage my home in Stuart. I've asked you to take a day or two away from Dad and stay at my place, but you turn up your nose. I've begged you to visit one of the boys, but you won't hear of it."

This afternoon Mom asked me if I thought we should put Dad in a Home. So that is her solution. His nastiness is almost unbearable. He wants everything on the double and raves until he gets his way. He is wearing the hell out of me.

I don't want to work here anymore. I'm frazzled with the worry of them both. I feel used. I cannot take it any more. I cook, clean, get him up, down, potty, dress him, take him on trips. And still Mom tells me what to do and how to do it. It has become a matter of power. We three seldom agree.

"Where two or three are gathered." Where are you, God?

Note: His power—screaming, rejecting.

Her power—caring for him, sitting with him, directing.

My power—bitching at both of them.

November 5, 1976

COUNTDOWN

'Tis bleak the day when father sits at home

His manly virtues we wrapped in baby's bib

And endless dribble from a mouth once shut

But now the man, full cycle back to crib.

Ah, beauteous heartbreak of a Mother's wiles

To serve the man she loves as servant bid

To bear the brunt of every helpless act

To be his crutch, though once carved from his rib.

Yet God is teaching us a lesson proud

"This way, my child, leads forward to the shroud

From dust to dust, from miracle to miracle

These moments glib but teach you to be bowed."

While life's vainglorious search leads ever onward

Yet wrapped within the Self a secret seed

Imprinted in the perfect divine pattern

From which evolves our individual creed.

MOM NEEDS A VACATION

November 16, 1976

Dad has improved. He is accepting his infirmity. He doesn't point to the arm and cry as he used to. He lies silently in bed waiting for breakfast. As I read late and am up many times for night duty, I try to sleep through the rattle of morning dishes. Mom makes the breakfast.

Living through last week was frightening. Anger covered my fear—anger at Mom's weakness, knowing she should get away. Knowing that I am so tired that I can hardly face dressing that man one more morning, and getting him to sit on the porch.

Mom and I discussed hiring a live-in aide to sleep with her in the other twin bed, but she doesn't want one. And I can't tear myself away from the injured man. He is part of myself—my body. It's as though I, too, were paralyzed, identifying with his illness. Underneath it all is fear, fear, fear. God has perhaps created this for a purpose: To teach me to serve. I rage inwardly at God.

Lately I have felt bitterness and resentment at my life's fading—a feeling of futility and hopelessness. I am like a fish caught in a net. I am only injuring myself being here with Mom and Dad, caught in the power conflict. I told Dad today that if he didn't stop yelling, he would have to go to a Home.

Mother's health is deteriorating. The doctor confirmed that she has had two mini-strokes this week. She needs quiet. She may have to go away.

December 10, 1976

DEATH'S ALTAR

To turn thus, silently to speak

And see my life, far-flung upon a shelf;

Dreams, hopes and wishes I did seek

Are lost in reverie within myself.

Have I with honor left them there

Or have I turned away from sorrow's door?

But see, the cupboard now is bare.

What remnants do I have of life's small store?

Shall I, by turning deep within

Give up the battle-chance to stay and fight?

How contact both these worlds and win?

Is there nowhere an answer to my plight?

The world is vast and strong my will

All things you wish can become manifest;

But turn the screw of thought and love

And dreams upon an altar you'll behest.

A QUESTION OF DIET

December 17, 1976

Today I launched into my health food argument for the hundredth time, urging Mom to drink low-fat or skim milk and go lighter on the salt. She's had high blood pressure and has only one kidney.

"Both of your sons drink skim milk. Perhaps they learned from Dad's stroke. Whole milk has fat which collects on the arterial walls, bringing on hypertension and eventually a stroke or heart attack," I preached, quoting from my classes in yoga with Swami Vishnu DeVenanda. "And salt in your diet is only asking for trouble, because it helps you retain fluids in your body which again leads to hypertension, disease and death!"

I was fighting for Dad's health as well as for hers.

"I've lived this long and I'm ready to go," Mother retorted. "I've eaten the same way for years and I'm not about to change. It was all right for my parents and it's all right for me."

"But your parents didn't have the foods we have today in the supermarkets," I argued. "Now canned goods contain preservatives and artificial colors, and animals are injected with chemicals that cause cancer. Why do you think Dad had his stroke? Don't you think it's partially what he ate all those years? And you still insist on giving him ice cream every night, whole milk, meat, eggs and salt! You're going to kill him with another stroke."

The argument is hopeless. She rages against me and insists I buy whole milk and give it to Dad. I buy both and slip him the light milk whenever possible.

"Doris, I just want to live long enough to outlive Dad so I can take care of him," says the lady who is my mother.

I can admire her for her persistence, if not for her intelligence, Dad's words ring in my ears, "Polly, you can't think." Dad, you were right. It's hard to change old habits.

GIFT OF LOVE

January 16, 1977

When I was six, I asked Mother to stop living her life through me, sensing even then that she communicated better with children than with her own husband. Perhaps I have been living my life through her, needing acknowledgment, love and understanding, needing someone I could trust. But somehow, somewhere, I turned off her love and stopped trusting her.

Perhaps that occurred when I was sent away at the age of four to visit an aunt in Chillicothe, Ohio. Upon returning home, I discovered that my baby brother, Robert, had been born. I felt then that I had been replaced and have been living out that lie ever since. Bob had Don, Mother had Dad and I had my cat.

This is part of my basic anger and jealousy in this new situation. I feel victimized and unacknowledged and am often angry at Mom.

I shared my emotions with a friend recently and she was upset. "Don't treat your mother like that, Doris. She needs kindness. She bears a lot."

"Too much," I retorted. "She won't let go. That's the problem."

Yesterday I took her for an X-ray of her spine. The doctor frightened me with, "I'm afraid your mother has cancer. It looks like it in these two ribs that are so thin."

I wouldn't believe it. Perhaps it was just a broken rib. But I was scared. "She won't let go, even for a day. She needs a rest and won't take one. It's hard on me watching her go. Can't you understand?" I unburdened myself, seeking some understanding and, perhaps, sympathy.

We will get another opinion.

I must grab hold of God within me and become dispassionate. I must turn and be cheery as we all go under. There is no death anyway—we only go to another state of change.

I mustn't fear or cling to this life. I, too, must accept and co-operate with the inevitable, as one can't function with best results for the patient when one is angry.

Perhaps I must just remove myself from the situation, get back on my own feet, cease to live my life through them.

February 6, 1977

ONWARD

This is the lull before the storm

This is the sail to the other side

This is the sea-capsizing boat

This is the soul—astir, afloat

This, oh this is towards

what we strive

This, the crescendo before

the end

This is the sunset

this, the bend

in the road

You cannot look back

You cannot look back

onward

onward

ever

onward.

NURSING HOME

March 5, 1977

For the past few weeks, I have watched my mother's once beautiful face become corroded with pain and anxiety. The flesh has evaporated around her cheeks, calves and thighs. She weighs only ninety-eight pounds. Her skin hangs loosely like an old crepe dress that has been packed tightly in a drawer. She must get away from this constant strain.

I feel as though I am standing on a broken piece of ice, floating away from both of them, drifting helplessly away from shore. I reach out to help my parents but can't touch them. Whatever I do or say seems to cause more unhappiness and dissension and I end up hating them both.

Don has been visiting and will leave tomorrow. I call him from my house in Stuart. "You must help me, Don. We must put Dad in a Convalescent Home today because Mother's health is breaking down and I can't bear to watch it any more. Dad is wearing her down with his constant demands and she is allowing it by doing too much for him. I'm desperate and can't take it any longer. I want to take my own life. You'll be leaving in a few hours and it will be too late. Mom will never listen to me. She trusts your judgment. It's now or never!"

Mother had been listening on the other phone and her voice cut in now. There was no fight left in her. "All right, I'll go. We'll meet you at the Home."

We pull up in front of a low, beige building. It looks harmless enough. Will it prove detrimental to Dad? He can walk quite well if we support his right arm to steady him. I pause in the sterile lobby, repelled by the wax plants and stiff unused couches and chairs, then follow Mom and Don to the main office, where a handsome middle-aged man greets us.

Don outlines Dad's condition in short sentences that end abruptly like an epitaph. The man's eyes don't meet ours as he proposes putting Dad in a single room.

"But who would ring the bell for him if he needs a nurse?"

I protest. "Who will watch over him or even speak to him?" My protests are to no avail; Dad will be put in a single room. Don is angry at the man's apparent lack of compassion and assails him:

"Sir, you may have authority but you don't seem to care. We have been telling you about our father and why we are putting him in here. A woman is sitting in front of you with suffering on her face and you haven't looked at her once. Is it because all you care about is money?"

Mother is shocked and embarrassed. I am grateful that my feelings have been expressed. The man apologizes and says the single room is all that is available but he is sure Dad will be well taken care of. His explanation stills our doubts and we agree to leave Dad here.

MOTHER FLIES TO TEXAS

March 7, 1977

Dad shed a lot of tears when we left him. After a few days, the tears disappeared but he has become uncommunicative. Mom has gone to Houston to visit her son and daughter-in-law. When she left, her face was aglow with expectation and relief.

My schedule is so busy now that I can only visit Dad for a few minutes a day. I'm studying English at Indian River Community College mornings, rehearse for "Fiddler On The Roof" at night and have just opened a studio for "Yoga and Art" in Stuart.

I placed an ad in a local shopper for an aide and finally hired a big kindly black woman named Meg. She works four hours a day, helping to feed him and taking him for walks. Towering above the frail figure of my father, she is personable, gentle and strong. Already Dad points to the cane with a grunt when she comes into the room.

Today she played dominoes with him, but it takes him a long time to make a move. He was much more aware several days ago and I am disturbed. Perhaps it is the tranquilizers they are giving him.

Tonight Dad pointed to a letter from Mom and cried. Some response, I feel, is better than none. She'll be back soon, I assure him, anxious that he doesn't get the impression that his stay here will be permanent.

CHURCH SERVICE

March 12, 1977

Today is Sunday and we took Dad into the dining room for church services. Dad cringed when he found himself surrounded by a sea of white faces and shriveled bodies. He soon lost himself in the hymns, however, singing along wordlessly, tears welling in his eyes.

While listening to the sermon, I thought of his contribution to the Congregational Church. As an elder, he was responsible for voting in three different ministers. I could picture him now—strong, dashing and silent, waiting to pass the collection plate, humility and pride mingled in service. "We give Thee but Thine own, whatever the gift may be. All that we have is Thine alone, a trust, Oh Lord from Thee."

That which we give will be returned to us, I thought, full-measured and running over. Watching Dad's tears of love, joy and sadness at his own limitations, I was glad that I had insisted he be taken to church. Although he loved life and nature more than people, he also loved to serve God. His gift to me was life. Serving him in his illness was a small sacrifice.

I left Dad briefly to call Mother in Texas. I wanted to prepare her for his worsened condition. "Mother," I exclaimed. "Dad has a large bump on his head. I don't know how or when he got it, but perhaps he fell out of his chair, as they've given him drugs and he is not tied to his chair. I just wanted to warn you that he isn't doing as well as when we brought him in here. It could be the medication, or depression. I just don't know."

She was concerned and immediately suggested taking an earlier flight home. Apologetic now, I urged her to stay. "You need your vacation. I just wanted to prepare you."

UNITY

March 14, 1977

Mother arrived from Houston and we brought Dad home today. After a week at the Convalescent Center, he is practically a bed patient again. He can barely walk, even with assistance. Mother flutters before him, uttering breathless little protests. "He can't walk. Don't walk him!" This only emphasizes his helplessness. Janice is heartsick, for all of her work must begin over again. Months of rehabilitation have been lost.

Now I know why the man at the Convalescent Home wouldn't look Don in the eye. They don't have enough aides there. One woman is assigned to fifteen patients. Overworked as they are, they get only $2.20 an hour. No wonder Dad had been ignored.

It will be a long time before we consider putting Dad into a nursing home again.

PRAYER

April 6, 1977

Mother wanted me to stay home tonight, as she doesn't feel well, but I had to go to church to pray for her health. Fear was invading every fiber and sinew of my being. I could not face the future of Mom's disintegration and Dad's worsened condition. I had to pray and become strengthened by positive thoughts. I need hope desperately—and health.

April 10, 1977

Dad is improving but Mom is getting worse. She is still

beautiful and strong but gets the "blind staggers" every week and has to lie down until it goes away. Her vision blurs. All this is the result of small mini-strokes or TIA's (Transient Ischemic Attacks). The symptoms generally last only a few moments but can persist up to twenty-four hours.

Warning signs include "dizziness or unsteadiness; a change in mental abilities; temporary numbness or weakness in the face, arm or leg; garbled speech or inability to speak; eye problems, like a sudden dimness of vision in one eye or tunnel vision; or recent severe headaches."

As I watch my parents' health rise and fall and old age approach, I look out at the Indian River and realize that it is spring again, one year after Dad's stroke. The water is ruffled with the remnants of strong winds from the North. The earth is dried and there are numerous brush fires around town. The wind probes the palm trees, knocking loose branches to the ground. The grass is white with frost and the air holds the chill of winter. It is difficult to believe that this is Florida.

Dad sits in his easy chair, looking at the passing scene. There is something here that God is working out: a family triangle of opposing powers—father, mother, and daughter. Holocausts of jealousy, anger, pride. Mother tries to help Dad get up and down. I prevent this to protect her. Dad rejects me. Tonight I sang "Ave Maria" in Mom's room. Dad wept.

WEAKENED LINK

April 29, 1977

Fear overcomes me when I realize how the three of us are dependent upon each other for survival. Tonight I called for Mom when Dad howled without letup. Although I've turned him over and given him his pills, the howling continues. It numbs my brain and I forget how to take off this dammed blue shirt, and how to put it back on.

It is 8:30 p.m. I think Dad is angry with Mom for reading complacently in bed. She is glad to get away and welcomes the respite. He has been in bed all afternoon. She still has not come in to say good night before he goes to sleep.

"Mother, will you please come in here!" I explode above his wounded howls. She is my life raft for the moment. She shuffles in wearing a faded flowered smock, irritated at the interruption and that she must leave her romantic novel. She is grateful for these few stolen hours earned because of her present pain and nervous condition. Dad quiets down although the room still rings with his persistent "Huh-huh-huh's." She tries to kiss away his bad mood.

My evening is a nightmare. As soon as I lay down on the floor to sleep on my cerise blanket, adjusting my pillow and pulling up the red plaid mohair, Dad moans. I have to get up slowly, crawling towards Dad's room on my hands and knees until the blood flows through my numb arms (I sleep with my arms over my head). I try to get to him before Mom wakes up and then return to sleep. Fifteen minutes later, Dad cries again. An hour later he whimpers and I have to give him his urinal. Ad infinitum through the night!

SHINGLES

April 30, 1977

Mom has shingles. She lies on her blue bed in her blue room dressed in a powder-blue nighty, her small frame diminished by pain. For the past three weeks, she has slept most of the day and night. She seems as fragile as an eggshell.

Her insistent threats and complaints: "I'll do it myself;" "Don't tell me what to do;" "Stay out of my kitchen;" "Go home! I don't need you here," have evaporated, along with her physical strength. I have witnessed the slow deterioration of her indomitable will.

"Why does this have to happen to me?" she asks weakly. "Why must I suffer so?" If the shingles, which started as an itching rash on her arm and chest, travel all the way around her body, she can die. Am I to be audience to this offending

stranger, Death? Although I have admired her fierce asser-
tion, "I will not let Dad go to a Home!" it has worked against
her. I have stood by helplessly as Dad's demands helped to
erode the substance and fiber of her life.

What can I do to alleviate her pain? Did I help to cause
it? I remember once when Bob stated fiercely, "Doris, you and
your eternal problems helped cause Dad's stroke." Stunned, I
reviewed my life. Dad had bought me my Spanish-style house
in Stuart ten years earlier. I was in show business and on the
road a lot. Now I had a place to come to between jobs, but when
I started to perform in Miami, the other jobs became fewer.
I missed the one-week stands and yearly bookings. Living in
a hotel and performing one show a week was not enough to
keep me occupied.

I finally moved to Stuart and stopped performing, making a living by teaching yoga and painting an occasional portrait. I had promised to pay Dad a percentage of the mortgage,
but never kept my word. My self-image was that of a starving
artist—in and out of work.

Perhaps I had been the dependent child, but now it was
my parents' turn to depend on me. It was my opportunity to
grow up and take responsibility. The feeling of being needed
was new to me and I often sank beneath the burden, or fought
loudly to be heard. Dad's health was my sole aim until Mom's
started to dwindle and then I had to balance my energies between the two of them.

I thought of Dad's wracking cough before breakfast (before his stroke) and the many times I had warned him, "Dad,
you're not getting enough oxygen. You should give up smoking, you know!" He ignored me and the only times he was
without a cigarette or pipe dangling from his lips was when
he ate, slept, or bathed.

"Stroke," I read in John Sarno's book, "is often the result of
a lack of oxygen in the brain cells." I, myself, had quit smoking after learning that my manager had died coughing in the
bathtub. I had been sufficiently frightened that I threw my

cigarettes out the window, never to smoke again. I could now sing without coughing. Food tasted better and I gained some weight, which I later fought against through yoga exercise. But I could breathe!

How right I had been when I tried to warn my father: "Please stop smoking, Dad, or you will pay for it." We are being sucked into his obit of pain and frustration—all because of one little cigarette.

READING ALOUD

May 10, 1977

Tonight Mother read aloud to Dad from "Captains and Kings" by Taylor Caldwell. She wears the green reading cap perched over her tousled silver curls. The skin of her lovely face, carved by pain and worry, is pulled taut and crinkled over her diminishing bony features.

She lay in bed later, one bare breast itching with pain. The light-blue gown was pulled from her shoulder, and shingles violated her shoulder blade. A pink and white symphony of weakening strength, she struggles to retain a last vestige of power, holding fast to the life in her man and the life within her own frame. Vaguely aware of her own ravaged flesh, she is conscious primarily of an ever-present weariness and the stark frustration of Dad's eternal "Huh-huh-huh's."

Yet it doesn't matter any more. Nothing really matters. She never listened to him when he spoke. Could she have helped to cause this? Why is it so difficult for people to communicate? And is it really so terrible for him? Exasperation and futile hopeless crying jags accompany his brief morning tantrums.

Morning. Mother enters Dad's room with a bright compassionate smile. She greets him with "Good morning, Bobby," as though he were a two-year-old, rather than a seventy-nine year-old man.

NEW ADDITION

May 22, 1977

On the way home from college in Fort Pierce (where I am taking a writing course to keep my sanity), I stopped at a produce market. There was no produce. Instead, a family of little kittens crawled around in empty wooden bins. A toothless, old Italian woman, stooped but spry and dressed all in black, was selling the remaining kittens.

A small boy held a tiny gray and white kitten upside down. "This one's mine," he exclaimed gleefully. The kitten was marked like "Muffin," a nine-year-old angora cat I grew up with as a child. Muffin had supplied many neighbors with kittens. I dared not ask the boy for his kitten, but searched the shelves until two gleaming yellow eyes in a soft gray body caught my eye. It was love at first sight.

"You would not dare keep me awake nights meowing under my window at three a.m, now would you?" I purred. She looked sweet and defenseless and I decided to take her home with me.

"Surprise!" I exclaimed, placing the tiny Persian newcomer on Dad's twin bed. Mom turned over slowly, groaning with pain. She froze in shock. Then a smile spread across her face.

"Oh, she's too cute not to ... " I held my breath for fear that she would not want a cat in the house. "To keep," she completed her sentence.

Thank God. I have a friend now. Something to love and be loved by. I shall call her "Hi-Tail," as she is always happy and walks with her tail straight up in the air. Perhaps she will bring a little joy into our lives.

Note: Mom's "cancer" was only broken ribs. I am relieved.

DOPE AND THE DOLDRUMS

May 29, 1977

Janice has worked with Dad for nine months. She has done a good job, but now seems to be wilting like a dying flower. I think the Nursing Home experience took the heart out of her. She sits around smoking and drinking Coke, when not helping Dad.

Arriving for breakfast, she exercises him, feeds him, bathes him, dresses him, plays dominoes and reads to him. But it is disheartening to help rehabilitate a man back to his feet and to have all your good work go for naught.

Mom's agony of the past few months has taken its toll as her flesh melts away. Her fighting spirit has been subdued by the shingles. She has laid in bed for one month now, her suffering eased by Quaaludes.

Mother does not want Dad to walk because he is so weak, but that is precisely why he should walk. I finally realize that it takes two people to walk him, one behind him holding on to the loop of his pants, and the other at his right side so he won't fall.

MOTHER'S COLLAPSE

May 30, 1977

Mother no sooner sat down to eat this morning when Janice looked over and said, "Polly, wake up. You're falling asleep over your breakfast."

Observing her half-empty coffee cup, I admonished, "Mother, Aunt Charlotte died after a cup of coffee, remember?" At that, Mom slumped to the side, and I reached out to catch her.

"Mother, Mother, wake up," I cried, but there was no response. Her face was white and immobile. My God, was she dead? Janice and I carried her to the couch and then I called the doctor.

"Bring her in at 9 a.m.," the nurse ordered. I called 911 and an ambulance arrived within ten minutes. Three men rushed in with a stretcher and gave her oxygen. They ordered me to find all her pills, the Quaaludes and Emperin III with Codeine.

"Mom, can you hear me?" I asked. "Do you hurt?" She screwed up her face and said in a quavering voice, "Dad!" Not "Bob," but "Dad."

I followed the ambulance to the hospital. "Acute gastritis and extreme exhaustion," the doctor explained. When I visited her later, she seemed happy and relieved to be in the hospital. "Oh, Doris, I'm so exhausted," she confessed. Great! At last she realizes it herself. This hospital stay is a God-send and will help alleviate the mounting pressure she has been unable to cope with since her illness. Letting go isn't easy, however. She told some visiting friends that she had to get out of bed to do "night duty."

She had a double room without a view, which even in her doped-up state made her unhappy. The next day she asked for and received a very nice single room overlooking the water. All is well, except that she seems to have lost her sense of time, getting breakfast mixed up with lunch.

I collapsed in the checkout line of a grocery store today, unable to walk and had trouble getting my breath. The terrified clerk called the manager who asked, "Do you want an ambulance?"

"Oh, please, no!" I said. "Both of my parents are already ill, one in the hospital and the other at home with a stroke. I can't afford to be sick. Just let me lie down and I'll be all right."

Forty minutes later, I was driven home to rest and told to recuperate. Dreamers! But I shall try to heed the warning.

June 1, 1977

THE CHOICE

When life hangs upon narrow thread

    Exhausted, one may wait for death

To dreams and hopes no longer wed

    From past experience now cleft

One waits, and silent, stirs the leaves

    Of memory—one thought may cleave—

            "Turn back:

"Turn back, turn back the wheels of time;

    I yearn to live. Give me a sign."

When withered body, broken mind

    Accepts the stranger, Death—alone

The battle rages, and we find

    Although we lie here, helpless—prone

A tiny seed, a flickering flame

    Cuts through the icy, gnawing pain

            "Turn back."'

"Turn back, turn back the wheels of time;

I yearn to live. Give me a sign."

MOTHER RECUPERATES

June 5, 1977

It's been a week since Mom got sick. This is a terrible night for Dad and me. I'm exhausted. What a time to be taking courses at Indian River Community College. I could not get one page of English Literature read before Dad called. I gave him Valium, a drink of water and turned him twice. He cries a lot. I suppose he is worried because Mom is in the hospital. It could be he needs more reassurance.

Janice is thinking about leaving and our new aide Dana alternated with her daughter today a lovely young black woman. They have both worked at a nursing home.

Mother called at dinnertime from the hospital and I let Dad listen to her. "How is Dad getting along without me?"

"He misses you, but knows you are well taken care of. We're glad that you can have a rest," I assured her.

I visited her in the morning. Seated alone in a corner, wan and diminished, she looked like a vanquished queen. I thought of her own regal mother, Grace Carpenter Rhodes (after Rhode Island) Moore, and of our ancestral heritage, which includes the brilliant martyr and author, Sir Thomas More. Must we all suffer in our own way?

"I thought you weren't coming," the small voice cried plaintively. "Please pass the pillow for my back." Her voice was high and reedy, as if too much fear and fatigue had damaged the windpipe. She looks better, but all she seems to care about is sleep. Strange turn of fate to have two parents down, leaving me among the ruins.

June 6, 1977

LAST RITE

I've but a day or so

before I go

A moment in a mile

A finger-full of fantasy

before I'm free

I've got a treasured

measure

of things I want to do

And things I must give up

before I sup

BLACK AND BEAUTIFUL

June 7, 1977

Janice has agreed that she needs a break. The job is long and wearing. She was one of our better aides, serving us well and willingly. Our new aide, Dana comes well recommended by neighbors. She is big, shiny-black and beautiful. The first day we walked Dad together. Now she can walk him alone. He has a good grip on the cane and she supports him under his right arm. Another miracle!

I have oodles of homework, an essay to write, chores to do and groceries to buy. God is good! I hope Mom will now realize she must live for herself first before she can assist another. It is a blessing to be able to help out in this situation. I feel wanted and needed, although it is difficult to watch your parents' power diminish. Every day has a different texture,

like the ocean waves. Yesterday I was ready to put Dad in
a nursing home because my efforts are not acknowledged. I
suppose parents feel about their children the way children
often feel about their parents—unappreciated.

At last, however, I am able to take some responsibility.

DOUBLE DUTY

June 8, 1977

Mother has come home and now I have two patients. I
wrap her in blankets and urge her to sit in my yellow easy
chair. After helping her dress, I then take her for a walk.

"You must help yourself get stronger by walking a little
more each day," I urged. "Mother, you are the patient now.
We've got to learn how to be our own person. Let God live in
you first, your husband, second. Doesn't the Bible tell us to
love ourselves first, and our neighbor as ourselves? You can
help Dad most when you stand up for yourself. Otherwise he
will moan and wail for attention only from you. If you give in
all the time and spoil him by treating him like a baby instead
of a man, you will kill yourself. And then you won't be around
to take care of him."

I walk her slowly around the back lawn, letting her lean
on me for support. This is a switch, for the backyard has so
far been Dad's beat. I think Dad is feeling good about himself,
knowing he is not the only one who is sick. He is definitely
glad Mother is home and has calmed down a little.

The weaker my parents become, the stronger I grow. Life
is a cycle.

THE REAPER

Yonder, just ahead

She picks a glowing rose of red

Never stops to keen

On moments she has seen

Never knowing, facing future

Willowy and strong

That her soul will

Be plucked from her ·

Ere long

"Don't worry love, I won't leave you,"

She claims to broken man

Yet she herself, diminutive

And fading fast

Is but a part of

Life's plan

And soon life's greatest gardener

Will stoop to pluck

What she gave up.

UNDERTOW

June 10, 1977

It's my turn to collapse with a cold and utter exhaustion. Poor Mom had to get up to tend me last night and Dad had to be turned over once or twice.

It's shameful to have to pay a woman $25 to come all night just to turn Dad over once. But we both are at the end of our rope. If Mom goes in to tend him, I wake up. Sleeping on the couch, I hear her door creak every time. Tonight I told Mother she needs a rest. She is skinny and disintegrating.

"So I'm skinny and disintegrating. Go home, Doris! Go live your own life," she urged.

"But how can I leave when I'm more worried about you than about Dad? Dad might live from three to ten years, but you're letting him kill you."

I am sick with despair. I don't know which way to turn. I need someone to talk to, but who? A minister ... sociologist ... social worker ... psychologist? Someone, anyone, who could help talk Mom into taking a rest. It seems that counseling would be of more value to the primary caregiver than to the patient. Perhaps we can change Medicare to accomplish this.

When I threaten to put Dad in a nursing home so she can take a vacation, Mom bristles like a porcupine, and accuses me of trying to run things again. God, please help us.

BROKEN VASE

June 15, 1977

Don has come. It is as though I had a beautiful vase, which has fallen, crashing, splintering into a million fragments. I could not hear it shattering all around me, echoing in a thousand chasms, in the darkness of a cave called Death. Don has come. He will help me to pick up the pieces. Help me to mend the broken vase of our lives. His broad objective view will help us see the Truth, so we can start to mend our ways again and set our lives in order. I slept tonight on a couch in the garage, falling asleep with no blanket. I woke up cold throughout my whole body. I did not know I was so tired. I am old. I am old. "I shall wear the cuff of my trousers rolled." (T. S. Elliott.)

I walk about wearing Mother's old white sweater, feeling just like her—diminutive, shrunken to a core. Mother still goes in to help dress Dad. It is the physical contact she needs, the mundane duties of life. You cannot feel you love Dad or he loves you if you remain a casual observer, talking nonsensical things.

The only thing that's real is prayer. Mother holds her hands tightly together, tension and anguish pouring through her in relief that Don has come. She admits she was so physically tired that she couldn't do anything, therefore the tears.

I feel the weight of the last months pressing upon me like a heavy mound of earth. Now the soil is breaking. I can eat again and look at the sun and let tears stream down my face. And kiss my cat.

June 27, 1977

My lesson remains unlearned. There seems to be no fruition of anything, only a bigger burden on Mother. I am more afraid each day. We must find help. We are like two sinking ships. If only she would let me take Dad for a ride or *do* something! I don't want to eat with them. I don't want to SEE them anymore. Don leaves tomorrow.

TO THE PARK

July 2, 1977

I'm on duty today, Saturday. I drove Dad to a park in Fort Pierce for a picnic lunch. It's so much easier without Mother around to distract him. It's difficult enough for me to figure out what he wants without another person clouding the issue. Dad and I never lose our tempers when we are alone together. He kept his head up a lot on the two and a half-hour excursion. He loves the park, the trees, and the narrow winding river.

When we returned, I walked him twice around the house and he copied a page of letters in his book, yelling the whole time. I pushed the rolling table over his chair so he could draw. He likes to trace animals and today used color on a lion. He also glued shells to some felt. I wish there were a ceramics or occupational therapy shop around Jensen Beach.

RESPITE

July 10, 1977

Mom flew to Don's for a brief vacation, leaving Dad with Dana, our aide, and me. Don called to say that Mother misses Dad so much that he is having a hard time keeping her there. Dana says Dad doesn't act too excited at the prospect of her return, but I firmly believe that he does not understand many words.

Don will go to Maine this summer. When we ask Dad if he wants to go, he shakes his head no. Since Dad is grounded, Mom and I will be also.

NIGHT TRIALS

August 29, 1977

My father is truly crazy today. I guess we are lucky there have been no mishaps because of his violence. At 1 a.m., Mother tried to cover Dad with a sheet and he rebelled, screaming like a banshee. His eyes were explosive, almost demonic. I knew that if she approached him in this mood, he would probably swing at her.

"All right," she threatened. "If you won't let me put this sheet over you, I'll close all the windows." She didn't want him to catch cold, but he was always warmer than her and when they slept together, he was comfortable with all of the windows open; whereas she was always cold and wanted them shut. Now his anger mounted to a crescendo and I was sure he would wake the neighbors. His voice lowered and gurgled, then jumped two octaves.

She opened the windows and again tried to put the sheet over him. He kicked it aside viciously, thrusting her arm away with a fierce growl. I stood silently in the doorway watching, enveloped in a warm rosy glow from my meditation. But then I became afraid he would hit her and decided to intervene. Opening a window wider, I announced quietly, "I guess he knows what he wants when he wants it." I shut Dad's door and guided a now docile Mother back to bed.

"I'll take care of him next time," I volunteered. Two minutes later he erupted, yelling angrily. I went in and turned on the light.

"What's wrong?" He continued to scream, pointing to the bathroom. I shut off the night-light and he turned over to go to sleep.

"Do you want some water?" I asked. He rolled back abruptly before I had a chance to raise the bed, grabbed the glass almost defiantly. He drank it down, and turned over again.

"I put a Valium here and filled your glass," I informed him after a trip to the refrigerator. "If you want it, you can get it! Here's the sheet if you need it." I folded the sheet so he could grasp the end with his good hand and pull it over himself.

At 5:30 a.m. he wanted the sheet pulled up. He had put his penis into the urinal. Our next step was to teach him to hang the urinal on the railing, and then learn to place it on the table as he used to do.

PART FOUR

ROAD TO
RECOVERY

(December 1977 – August 1979)

Reaching the Plateau!

It is twenty months later. Mr. T has reached a "plateau", in his walking, exercises, and speech. We drive him to the beach and shopping, so Home Health care service has ended. Due to their faithful assistance, Dad now walks — almost, alone. He still needs round the clock care. Mrs. T has lost thirty pounds. Doris twisted and injured her knee and has been on crutches for several months now. But the Miracle of Mr. T. remains.

For Dad has been enjoying his home, the daily view of our long, sloping lawn to the river where he can watch sailboats, birds, and reflected sunsets.

11/7/77

We are learning to cope with his illness.

IV

RELATIONSHIPS

December 18, 1977

There is a sweetness between Mom and Dad that I don't recall seeing before, brought on apparently by their changing relationship. Before she had depended on him; now he needs her. "The mountains shall be leveled and the valleys filled," I thought once again. I am again shut out, but it's all right. They have lived their lives together and now their lives are nearing a close. Although we don't know which one will go first, we do know that the "stranger" is near, that he has struck several blows.

God puts us to bed tender. This sweetness I feel is shown in the way Dad wants her with him most of the time. Like a moth basking in the flame of her light, Dad absorbs her love like a child accepts the love of its mother.

While he still often wails and berates her, he is at other times cooperative and visibly grateful, loving to be kissed, caressed and catered to. "Grow old along with me, the best is yet to be ... " perhaps refers to life as it nears its end, for when we are forced to narrow our needs and wants to the barest necessities for survival, we find the things that mattered before become as transient shadows.

When Mother was unable to keep accounts, Dad cut her down. Now when I cut her down for the same reasons, he rages at me. When the daughter calls the mother "stupid" for such things as not taking a name and number over the phone; forgetting to note expenditures on the "out" side of a checkbook, etc., the tables have turned. His anger, which I used to resent, I can now forgive, for I recognize what traits in Mother drove him into violent temper tantrums. Now, when I reprimand Mother in front of him, he defends her.

PILLOW FIGHTS

January 5, 1978

We are fighting over pillows. Somehow they have come to symbolize validation, love, respect and acceptance. In reality, they are simply tools to make it easier for Dad to get up from chairs by himself.

All the chairs in the house are too low for him because of his very long legs. If we could adjust it so that he could get up without help, it would make it easier for all of us.

It's exasperating to always have to be there to help him do something as simple as rising from a chair. But then, even if he gets up alone, one of us has to help him adjust his sling and button or unbutton his sweater. I have learned a couple of useful tricks. If I stand to the side and use my middle finger to gently press him forward two or three inches, he can put his good hand on the arm of the chair and push himself erect.

Here is where an Occupational Therapist would come in handy, but there doesn't seem to be one near here. I want to take him to the Rehabilitation Center in Palm Beach, but Mother doesn't think he should be driven that far. And she's the boss. Dad takes her side, reinforcing my feelings of rejection.

One day I covered a foam cushion and slipped it under the pillow on his easy chair. He sat down and realized he was higher. In two seconds he popped up, ripped out the offending pillow and slung it across the room. Then he sat down, satisfied. I was astonished. Amazing! He was able to stand alone in anger to remove a pillow only to sit down and play the dependent child, exhorting us to help him up again.

How can you reason with a stroke patient? You can't. You have to enter their mind and realize that they are terribly threatened by being so helpless and this fear leads to anger at their situation. They use this sense of dependency to make sure they won't ever be left alone. It becomes a security blanket. But if we are overprotective, that blanket can become a tomb, for in smothering them with attention they may become permanently crippled, their initiative stunted.

"Dad," I tried to reason. "You just got up by yourself, which proves that if you get mad enough you can do it! Why not use the pillow and become independent? You can learn to stand by yourself and walk to the door, going out and coming back eventually by yourself if you want to. It's all in your mind."

He raved continually during my whole speech. He does not want to do it himself. Perhaps he senses that Mother is afraid for him to do things alone because he may fall again. After all, he has fallen several times so far—on the grass, on a tile floor and in the living room with Mother.

When Mother fell with him, she reported: "We went down together. He lost his balance and fell almost on top of me but no one got hurt." Thank God. And here I am trying to help him become more self-sufficient while walking and hoping he can get up from his easy chair by himself.

Today I tried to hide the pillow beneath his cushion again. He raved until I helped him up to remove it. And when Dad yells, the neighbors know it! It is difficult to play the role of disciplinarian with Mom standing by ordering me to get him up.

This incident so upset me that I removed all of the furniture and plants from the front porch, leaving Dad's chair (to which I had attached three pillows firmly with string), and Mother's cushionless low, white chair. Determined to teach Dad how to be independent, I walked him down the ramp to seat him in the pillowed chair. He sprang up like a rocket and

plopped down in the low chair before I could stop him. He
would not budge. Mother took the high chair.

"Whatever happened to all the porch furniture?" she
asked innocently. I sat in silence on a folding chair, glaring at
my belligerent father, my blood pressure slowly rising. Foiled
again! All of the furniture was locked in my van and now I
needed a derrick to get Dad out of the low chair.

There must be some way to have a "win-win" situation,
but so far I have not found it. Reflecting upon our behavior, I
realize that all of my life my mother tried to help me out of
every difficulty. She even found the house in Stuart and urged
Dad to buy it for me. While on the road in "Show business,"
I had stored my belongings in Boston and Chicago. When I
found out that my clothes had been stolen, I decided to find a
permanent place of my own.

Isn't there a parallel here? Just as Dad tried to support
me by letting me do things for myself, so I am trying to help
him get up and walk alone. Mother's desire to help, although
she meant well, can be detrimental in the long run. For one
serves another best by helping him become independent. I
may love being taken care of, but when they tell me what to
do, I rage. Allowing them to make choices for me dulls my
ability to make my own decisions.

I now realize that Dad's lack of support when he and Mom
argued over how to help me was due to his desire for me to
gain independence. At the time, I had misjudged him, reading it as a lack of love. In the same way Dad is angry with me
when I try to get him to help himself. He probably feels I am
rejecting him.

THE CHILDREN'S HOUR

March 10, 1978

I have been feeling sad and inadequate that I am unable
to find any interesting activities for Dad to do with his good
left arm. It's been two years now since his stroke. Although

he has progressed from denial and depression to anger, I have had visions of him standing before his workbench in the garage. But what can he do with one arm, especially since he has to hold on to a cane to keep his balance?

In spite of my two years experience in the Women's Army Corps as an occupational therapy assistant, I am still unable to come up with any ideas. I bought him a book of animal drawings which he enjoyed tracing with his left hand. Although slow and painstaking, at times he would give a whoop of delight. The roaring lion was his first choice. Apropos! An attempt at painting by numbers was a complete flop and he showed only a mild interest in finger painting. Gluing shells onto a white Styrofoam Christmas tree was our most successful venture, although I did most of the gluing.

I have been taking courses in English, journalism and speech at Indian River Junior College and recently signed up for a course in children's literature. I had hoped to study pre-school stories, since I write and illustrate for this age, but the course covered pre-teen literature, which didn't interest me.

While reading "Robin Hood" for class, however, I thought that the story might appeal to Dad. It's been difficult finding books that interest him. He dismisses mysteries, romances or any complicated subjects. "Robin Hood," however, was a hit and we followed with "The Little Prince," "Heidi," and "Treasure Island."

In reading to Dad every evening, we have been able to relive our own childhood. A wealth of emotions wells up within me, and many times I am too choked up to continue. I look up at Dad and he, too, is smiling through his tears.

This has opened up another means of communication in addition to singing, which Dad loves to do. He can carry a tune and harmonizes very well, without words. As we read to him, however, he weeps and laughs at all the correct places, which never ceases to amaze me. When the speech teacher visited us, Dad could not point to a knife, dog, key, or spoon.

How on earth can he understand the words in a story when he can't associate the word with the picture?

When Dad gets tired of our reading, he asks for the book and shuffles through the pages until he finds the end of a chapter. Stop here, he'll gesture with a few "Wa-wa-wa's." Well, if he is happy and seems to understand, that, in itself, is progress!

CHURCH VISITOR

April 16, 1978

I called the church a week ago and spoke with the minister's wife, explaining our trials and anguish. I asked for help.

"Dad sits alone in the backyard by the hour. He has no one to talk to, and the house is overrun by females. I really feel he would profit by having men visitors now and then. We have friends, but it is difficult for them to see him like this. Do you have any suggestions?"

Mrs. Polheim, a warm and supportive woman, promised to see what she could do. As Dad was on the board of deacons for many years, I supposed some of the men might come to our rescue.

Today Mr. Lewis stopped by. He is a likable, heavy-set gentleman with two chins and a big belly. He and Dad are carrying on a one-way conversation in the backyard about the weather, the news, and the church. I can tell from Dad's occasional "Wa-wa-wa's" that he is very happy to see his friend. He is following every word and trying his darndest to communicate with a head shake and facial muscles. Off and on he will close his eyes and let his head nod, then comes to and acknowledges his visitor with a half smile.

Mr. Lewis is suggesting that Dad go to church and I think that this is just the encouragement that Dad needs, for whenever I suggest we go, Mother says no. Perhaps she is afraid he will cry. But if he does, so what? I feel in my heart that Dad would enjoy church immensely. After all, isn't this the very time when one needs a strong relationship with God? Perhaps if he goes a number of times, the emotional stress will lessen. I am grateful to Mr. Lewis for inviting us to go, as now maybe Mother will cooperate.

DAD GOES TO CHURCH

May 30, 1978

We have taken Dad to our church several times. At first, he cried aloud and we had to take him out. Finally, the three of us began sitting in the back. Mother can't hear the sermon from the back because she is partially deaf, but won't go down front alone, preferring to stay with Dad. We are beginning to become acclimated. We take Dad out before the service is over.

PAPA'S CHOICE

June 2, 1978

For several months now, salesmen have visited the house to show Dad a new car. He has not approved of any of them, thank God, as Mother ordered two doors and our old Chrysler is a four-door. I don't know why Mom wants a two-door, as we already have a two-door Anglia Ford to run around in.

Dad has been very upset and is often rude to the smiling salesmen. He roars and shakes his head no. Often he will not step into the car without a great deal of persuasion. I am beginning to wonder if he and I do not agree that we need a four-door, which I can drive to Maine. I want to be able to carry passengers and luggage, and sleep on the road when necessary. Besides, the little cars are difficult for Dad to sit in comfortably as he is over six feet.

Perhaps Dad is resenting our putting him in the back seat while Mom and the driver sit up front. Whatever, I am unable to get Dad to communicate why he is so adamant against buying a new car.

Today the three of us drove to a Chrysler-Plymouth dealer. As we walked into the showroom, I noticed a beautiful beige and blue four-door. Charlie, the redheaded salesman who has served us all these years, gave Mom a big smile and ignored Dad. I guided him to a chair.

Charlie began to point out the two-door at Mother's request. Dad sat on the edge of his chair, wobbling his cane and shaking his head. He obviously wanted to go home even though we had just arrived. Charlie's smile soon diminished when he saw that Dad wanted to leave and he led Mom into a hallway. I followed and overheard his words.

"Mrs. Thurston, I would suggest you pay no attention to your husband. He probably doesn't understand anyway. After all, he isn't going to be driving—you will."

"But I do want him to like it," she protested.

I stepped in to defend Dad. "Charlie, no way am I going to let Mom buy a car Dad doesn't like. He knows what he wants and it's probably a four-door. Dad is perfectly sane. He has aphasia and he is unable to talk, but we just haven't found the right car yet. It's important to encourage stroke patients to make decisions and to include them in family decisions.

"We're really looking for a bucket swivel seat so we can get him in and out of the car easily," I went on. "Dad's tall and needs lots of leg room. Mom's short and needs to sit farther forward to drive."

Charlie's face brightened. "Then why not look at the Plymouth Fury. You can push both seats back because they move separately."

"Let's try it, Mother," I urged. "It's important to please Dad. Just because he can't talk doesn't mean he can't reason or decide. It seems to me he is still head of the house and we should let him have a choice in the matter."

I returned to Dad and began helping him up. "We're going to look at a four-door, Dad. Let's see if you like it. We'll all go for a ride and then we can decide."

He grunted "Huh-huh-huh," nodded in agreement, and we shuffled towards the door. He looked pleased as he paused to take in the sleek car. Charlie helped him into the front, adjusting the seat so his legs would fit comfortably. Mom and I sat in the back, enjoying the plush blue-gray upholstery as Charlie took us for a drive.

The atmosphere gradually brightened as each of us fell in love with the mechanical animal. Dad laughed at the air conditioner, a feature Mom had never been allowed to have in the past twenty-five years of Florida heat. He used to shake his head at Polly's "frivolity" in even suggesting it. What a difference a stroke makes, I thought.

The Fury had all the trimming, but what was more important, it had separate seats so Dad could move back and Mom could move forward. And it had a radio for me. We were all ecstatic and it was a sale. Charlie beamed as he helped Papa out of our new car.

This time his broad smile was for Dad.

FLOWER THERAPY

June 3, 1978

I tried flower therapy today while Mother went to the hairdressers. It was good to have a block of time in which I could be creative with Dad—alone. For if Mother were here, he would give all his attention to her. After setting out a card table in front of his easy chair, I brought out several vases, two of which he had made in ceramics. I then went outdoors to cut flowers and selected an assortment of purple, orange and crimson blossoms, adding leaves and dried sprigs, and laid them on the table before him.

"Now, Dad, how would you like to choose a vase?" He looked at me with a pained expression, gazing helplessly at the vases. I picked up a long-stemmed purple flower.

"Select a vase for this flower. Which one would you choose?" He reached for a slender double-curved blue vase and plunked the flower into it.

"Good. Now what else should you put with it?" Slowly he

began to sort and choose flowers and sprigs until he was satisfied with the effect.

"Beautiful," I exclaimed, picking up the vase to view the design from several directions. "Now where do you think it should go?" He pointed to the hall table and I placed it next to the Japanese doll. Mother returned as I was cleaning up. She looked perplexed.

"What's going on here?' I felt like a kid cheating in school.

"Dad created a flower arrangement. How do you like it?"

She looked at the lovely decoration and dutifully acknowledged his handiwork. I wondered if she understood my joy and feeling of accomplishment. This was not like dominoes, which Dad never tires of playing, yelling uproariously when he wins. Flower arranging, however, is a subtle art combining man's talent and God's beauty. Dad had, after all, planted the flowers and created the vase.

"Wonderful, Bob, dear," Mother exclaimed again, more joyously this time. Her kiss, planted on his forehead, was the perfect completion to our artistic venture.

WEEDING

June 4, 1978

Dad loves gardening. Could I entice him to help me weed? Today I placed his wheelchair next to the flowerbed in the backyard and proceeded to weed. After he observed me, pointing out what I should pull next, I casually suggested he help me. He pulled a few blades of grass and we felt we had done a good job.

I never appreciated how much effort goes into keeping up a place like this. Even though we have a man to cut the lawn, Dad spent a good portion of his time trimming, weeding, and planting. Just to keep the palm fronds picked up from fifty trees is in itself a chore.

I can imagine that Dad really feels quite helpless with

his useless right arm. No movement has returned to it even though we continue his daily exercise. Every time we acquire a new aide, I teach her the physical therapy routine. Sometimes Dad balks a little and we do what we can.

The morning routine:

1) Wash his face. This can be difficult as neither Mom nor I know if the other has done it. If Dad screams and points to the door, we don't know whether he is trying to tell us that's it's already been done, don't do it, or I want my breakfast.

2) Breakfast in bed.

3) Exercise in bed.

4) Bathroom.

5) Bathe him in bed.

6) Dress him.

7) Walk him into the living room and seat him in his easy chair.

8) Give him the morning paper.

No one is able to tell if Dad can read or not, although we think he can read numbers because he turns immediately to the stock market page and reads his investments. Sometimes we read him the funnies, which he seems to understand and enjoy.

GIFT OF LOVE

June 5, 1978

Because I could not give Dad what I thought he lacked, some kind of activity to wile away the hours, something he could create, do or learn, which would build his self-image, I finally, in desperation, asked God what I could do. "Perform," was the answer.

"But I can't perform for Dad! What do you mean perform?"

"Perform," I heard again. It's true, I thought. I can perform. It's the best thing I do—perform, and paint.

"But perform for whom?"

"Perform," my inner voice repeated. Then I shall perform for the old and infirm in nursing homes, I decided. I will bring to them the love I cannot give my own family. I recalled the many years of performing in nightclubs, churches, schools, theaters and the many kinds of audiences I entertained with song, dance, art and comedy. Why wouldn't the elderly also enjoy my acts? They were merely my former audiences grown up—or older.

I rehearsed "Portraits in Song" with a duo, which played violin, accordion and piano. My act included a medley of French songs from "Can-Can." We performed at Easter Manor in Ft. Pierce. I was shocked at the smattering of applause, then realized I was mistress of ceremonies, and hurried back to get a hand for the band. Afterwards I mixed with the audience and was surprised to realize that they really appreciated our show. The deaf, blind, sick, senile and the sedated. They commended me for my energy and love.

The cycle is complete. The gift of love has returned to itself.

BORTZ SPRING LAKE

June 13, 1978

We so enjoyed our performance in Fort Pierce that I decided to perform again for a nursing home in Hobe Sound, inviting a talented singer to join me with her medley of songs. "Jo" has had asthma for two years and had been unable to sing. I hope this will be a breakthrough for her and she will be able to sing again. She has a wealth of charisma and healing power in her voice and has sung in nightclubs, churches and prisons.

My act includes song, dance, art, and comedy in a condensed version of "My Fair Lady," in which I sketch a portrait of a patient while I'm singing. Jo and I closed the show with a duet.

Our show was a great success. Mother and Dad were in

the audience and Dad seemed to enjoy it. We were asked back to entertain again. My portrait model was a 97-year-old "lady killer" with a yellow hat and white mustache. Spry and very deaf, he had to be forcibly removed from the model stool. He could not understand that this was the end of the show.

Jo's voice was powerful and she sang more songs in the ward after the show. She will return with her son to sing again. I feel happy and fulfilled. I feel "me" for a change. My joy is to give joy and it comes back full-fold and running over. Perhaps God is trying to tell me something.

After the show, a glowing, voluble woman in a wheelchair clasped me to her bosom in a joyous bear hug. "Your show was wonderful," she exclaimed, "and it wasn't even religious!" I gather they have a lot of religious singing here. I can sense a lack of live entertainment in nursing homes from our experience so far. Here is a ready made audience for newcomers or for retired veterans in theater, music, dance, drama, etc. to practice on and share with. By giving we receive. It is more rewarding than working in nightclubs, as these people are shut-ins who see the same rooms, the same faces, day after day. How many bored retirees would come to life just by sharing their interests, talents and time.

I am again made aware of the fact that stroke patients (there were three in our audience) need to see new faces. If homebound, they need to get out of the house. It is important to bring outsiders into the nursing home, or bring a patient to a new environment, whether a church, a store, a museum or a beach.

My inner voice had born fruit, as the two musicians who played for me at Easter Manor visited Dad last Sunday, bringing us a concert of classical music and old songs. Dad joined in with gusto, carrying the melody and harmonizing with his "Wa-wa-wa's." Jo and I have been able to give of our talents, and the musicians will bring their piano, violin, and accordion to Bortz Spring Lake. Dad's need has touched many lives.

JOB OFFER

June 14, 1978

This morning I received an unexpected phone call.

"Doris, this is the Activity Director at Bortz Spring Lake. I am leaving tomorrow and we will need an activity director. Would you be interested in filling in until we can find someone to work steady?"

My heart sank. My God, to have to watch those old folks shuffle past my desk day after day! I had taken a brief tour of the home last night. Had they been preparing me for this?

"It was a truly enlivening experience to perform for them last night," I began, "but to come back there and work, even part-time, would be ... depressing, even frightening. I don't know if I could do it," I confessed. How could I live with those pale, white faces and disintegrating bodies day after day?

Never will I forget my arrival the previous night. Every resident was lined up along the hall for a fire drill—the deaf, the blind, the senile, the sick, and the aging. Here was a segment of society I have never had the opportunity to be with, except for my short visits with Dad at the Convalescent Home. Even then it had been a terrifying blow to the psyche, dwindling one's life force.

To be surrounded by the aged and dying is a shock because one is suddenly acutely aware of one's own mortality, knowing that Death lurks inside the vessel of our own bodies. It is all just a matter of time.

"All it takes to do the job is a lot of love," the girl stated. "I know you have worked in hospitals before and this won't be too difficult. You'll get the knack of it. If you'd like to come over, I can give you a tour and explain your duties, and then you can think about it."

"All right, I'll come. But I'm not promising anything."

I considered her offer. I knew nothing about being an activity director, but here was an opportunity to expand my awareness of the aged in my new career as aide and coworker with my father, preparing me, perhaps, for a time when I might have to put my own parents into a nursing home. The experience might help me care for Dad. Should I turn down an offer, which was the result of my "gift of love?"

TOUR OF BORTZ

June 15, 1978

I took the Bortz tour today. It was all so strange, even frightening. Perhaps I was haunted by memories of working with mental patients in army hospitals. It is horrifying to see what will happen to us when we get old. White faces and wizened bodies without names or memory. As I talked to the residents, however, I began to see them as valuable human beings. Perhaps it will be love that makes it bearable, for the spirit knows no age.

Visiting patients on the Medicaid wing was depressing. I did not relish walking down this hall. Is it because the quality of the aides is poorer or because patients are on more medication? They sit silently around tables in the dining hall like dead people. There is no communication. It is like a dream world. One or two seem alive and human—Sally, for example, whose ample body and young spirit are confined to a wheelchair, and the very acid Tina (who used to be a school teacher). Tall, lanky and distinguished looking, Tina's sharp inquisitive nose misses nothing.

"Are you going to work here?" she asks. "We could stand some action around here. These people are all dead or crazy." She looks around at the still bodies as if they were her students, and she was unable to rouse them.

I discover a lady eating with her fingers. She has delicate features, high cheekbones and an aristocratic nose. Her fingers are sensitive and aware as they search for food on her tray. The white hair is bobbed and wavy. Suddenly an unearthly scream echoes down the hall.

"Why is that baby crying?" asks the blind lady, deeply

concerned. Even her voice holds compassion and intelligence. The room fills with titters.

"That's another patient down the hall, Johanna," the nurse explains, beckoning me to follow her. We approach a woman, a once-famous writer, now shrunken, twisted and wild-looking. She is tied to her chair.

"I hear you were a writer," I said, handing her my pad and pencil. She howled, clutched the paper and tried to eat it. I withdrew in shock.

"Don't mind her, Doris," the nurse said, and turned to a diminutive old lady. "And this is Jane, a sweet lady. She is 90 years old." Jane's face is round and virginal, holding no trace of age. Her skin glows like a Dresden doll. Her fine, white hair is pulled tightly into a bun at the nape of her neck. Her body folds like a wilting flower, head resting over the chair arm. She is sleeping. The nurse slaps her cheek gently to waken her.

"Jane, Jane wake up. You have a visitor." The blue eyes open and look at me vacantly. "Jane worked once as a maid for royalty and look at her now! She's a good patient, though." No wonder she is a favorite. Her face is like a pale, white rose tinged with pink. We grow old in so many ways, I thought. What will my end be?

ACTIVITY DIRECTOR

June 30, 1978

After two weeks, I finally accepted the position at Bortz Spring Lake Nursing Home. The pay is ridiculously low, but I don't dare ask for more until I know I can do the job. I felt quite guilty thinking of all those patients without an Activity Director.

From my desk in the hall (I have no office), I can observe the residents in the dining room and greet them as they walk to their rooms. One favorite, "Mr. Woody," is an elderly blind man in his eighties. He is kind, considerate and humble. His faith, like Johanna's, the blind lady, is honed to a fine edge.

He knows that God has allowed him to live for a purpose, and everyday he prays to do His will. Awakened at 6 a.m., he listens to news on the radio. Al, his roommate, is a stroke patient confined to a wheelchair. Al acts as his eyes, telling Woody where his things are, and opening and closing doors for him. Often depressed, as are many stroke patients, Al has no family to visit him, whereas Woody is allowed to visit his daughter every weekend.

"It gets very lonely and boring sitting here in the morning before breakfast and at night after dinner," said Woody. "I'm glad you're here. We need more activities. We need visitors. I try to do my part and talk to people, but I can't get around too well, being blind. Al helps me by guiding me to meals. I hold on to his wheelchair and walk behind him."

I decide to look for a volunteer to read to Woody, Al, Johanna and Kaye, another middle-aged stroke victim whose faith is strong. Overweight, she is confined to a wheelchair. These four are keenly aware and should enjoy group discussions and inspirational readings.

I have been making the rounds every day. I finally realized that it is not only exhausting, but also useless to try and establish a rapport with several of the worst cases. I have all I can do as a part-time worker (three days a week) to keep the mobile residents busy.

Several activities have been set up already, including Bible study class and a monthly birthday party, when churchwomen come to sing and visit. In Bible study, I encourage the class to ask questions and share their views. If we are to know, respect and love one another, we must communicate.

I have started a morning session, which includes singing, games and sharing. I throw a large, light ball to everyone, then lead them in hymns. I often ask questions about the meaning of words before we sing them. In chair exercises, I incorporate a few moments of yoga breathing, relaxation, and some meditation. Residents' ages vary from fifty and up. Some are physically ill with bright minds; some are old, senile and silent; some are angry but attentive; some need sedation more than the others do.

I am getting to know my patients and to love them. Each is a distinct personality. One woman is very deaf. Her age is debatable, as she always adds several years, so we will complement her on how beautiful she looks at eighty-six, when the records say she is eighty-three. She is missing one leg below the knee and uses a wheelchair to get about. An independent character, she dresses herself in bed without any help and takes pride in her accomplishments. Her frame of wavy, white hair sets off a square, determined jaw.

Always perfectly groomed, she visits the beauty parlor in the home regularly. When we have activities in the dining room and there is to be music, she requests a front seat near the piano, where she hunches in her wheelchair and lifts her quavering voice in song. In my morning classes, I can tell when she is uncomprehending by the wounded look of isolation on her face. I then try to make her feel included.

"I used to play the organ for our church," she mentioned proudly the other day.

"Wonderful. Why don't you try to play us a little tune?" I asked, pushing her towards the piano.

"No, no. Don't you see I can't play, now? Look at my hands. They are all gnarled with arthritis. I couldn't possibly." She pushed herself away from the piano as if it were a poisonous snake.

Carl is in his seventies and is allowed to roam the grounds by himself. Although his sight and hearing are greatly impaired, he often sits with us, watching through thick glasses. Suzy, a plump lady who rarely talks—probably because she, too, is very deaf—pointed out that she needs glasses, but can't afford them. I am told the Lyons Club collects discarded glasses, so I shall bring in some for her to try—until I can do better.

Every morning and afternoon I must do a sales job, rounding up thirty people to attend activities, stimulating and motivating them. Helena, a delightful lady from Boston who treats her room like an office, storing letters and magazines in boxes, is definitely not a joiner.

"Oh, I have so much to do today. I am way behind on my correspondence and I have work that must be done. But if there's anything I can do for you, please tell me. We're so glad you're here. You mean a lot to this establishment. Keep up the good work."

I feel as if I am her employee. She did run an office and had much to do with Women's Rights. Helena is a comfort and a continual source of information as to what is going on in the Home, offering the latest tidbit of gossip.

I have sent for more "Talking Books" to see if Woody will use a record player. We can get "books," tape recorders, and record players from Daytona Beach, for anyone who is blind or disabled. I must write for information to "Talking Books, Library of Congress, Washington DC," to order a record player for Dad.

I am building up classes at Bortz. Several ladies from Hobe Sound have volunteered to teach sewing. Indian River Community College will send us a weekly slide show, a ceramics teacher and a "bird lady" who will show slides and play birdcalls on tape.

A woman has volunteered to meet for discussion with my special four, and another lady will lead singing (acappella), on Fridays. I invited a new minister to the home to give a sermon. Reverend Coombs was so upset by the experience that he decided to send a substitute the following week, hoping he might not have to come back. By the end of the month, however, he was hooked.

"I really enjoy preaching to these elderly people almost better than preaching in my own church," he confessed. "It's a challenge. They are so open and appreciative and full of love. I learn from them to be myself, which strengthens me to face my own congregation."

Reverend Coombs later brought his wife, who played the

piano and shared their children with us. The presence of a baby brings renewed interest in life to our "family."

DAD VISITS BORTZ

July 4, 1978

I invited my parents to join Bortz Spring Lake residents for a picnic on the Causeway. I had described Woody, Kay, Johanna and Sally, and was glad for Dad to have the opportunity to meet the residents. Mrs. McCathern, head of the Nursing Home, suggested I bring him in to meet her, and she would give me an evaluation of his illness. We are wondering if he will ever learn to talk again.

Dad lumbered down the hall to her office with his cane, and she invited him in to sit down. Observing his paralyzed arm, which is flaccid, immobile and bent inwards, she said matter of factly, "I am quite sure it will never come back. But," she added, "if you practice speech every day, I think you can learn to talk again."

Naturally, Dad cried. I excused myself to look for Johanna, hoping she would help to divert his tears. I pushed my blind patient into the room in her wheelchair. Frail and stoop-shouldered, her straw-colored hair framed the delicate face with the straight nose, a legacy of her German background.

"Dad, say hello to my favorite patient," I exclaimed. Dad looked at her through his tears and I placed her hand in his good one. He stopped crying.

"Johanna, this is my father. He's had a stroke and he can't talk. Dad, Johanna is blind, but she's my best patient and does morning exercises better than anybody else."

Only recently I had suggested that Johanna be moved to another room with a caring roommate. The nurse followed my advice and Johanna has four roommates and eats in the main dining room, where a kind black man with one hand and good eyes can help her locate her food.

Our visit was over and Mrs. Mac knew more about why

I took the job, and also why Dad is my first priority. I suddenly wondered if Dad's tears were because he feared we were thinking of admitting him here. Many times when I lost my temper I had threatened to put him in a Home. I had never really considered Bortz, however, as I know that he needs too much special attention. I don't believe he would be less depressed, but possibly more. And possibly less motivated, as he has never been a social creature.

FIRST SHOWER

September 5, 1978

After hiring a dozen or so aides this year, we finally hit the jackpot. Carrie, a towering motherly blonde who came to us through a nursing agency, took one look at Dad lying in bed this morning and asked, "Has he had a shower yet?"

"No," I admitted sheepishly. "We weren't sure of the technique and we didn't want him to fall stepping into the shower stall."

"Well, let's try it," she suggested. "It's really quite simple. It will save time and energy over giving him a bed bath. "

She asked Dad if he would like to have a shower and his eyebrows lifted in anticipation. Hurray! Carrie took off his pajamas and put on his new maroon robe and the old brown slippers.

Dad embellished his cooperation with eager "Ho-ha's." I fetched a stool and placed it inside the shower stall, covering the seat with a towel so he wouldn't slip when he sat down.

"Now, Mr. T, I'll take off your robe and we'll help you into the shower," Carrie said cheerfully. Letting go of the cane, Dad clung to the shower door and stood there, long, lean and naked. Carrie removed his left slipper.

"Now step up and over with your good left foot," Carrie ordered. "Watch this," she commanded. I watched as she placed her toe on the back of his right slipper. Dad pulled his foot out, grabbed the soap and dragged his weak leg in after him. Carrie helped him to sit down.

"It's much safer to hold on to the slipper and he just slips his foot out," she explained. "Then you're free to support him if he falls." Tricks of the aide! How simple it is once you know what to do. Bless people like Carrie, and all the aides and nurses who help us with our loved ones, for their knowledge gives us the assurance to carry on.

As Dad panted in anticipation, Carrie turned on the water taps, letting him adjust the temperature. Then she scrubbed his back.

"Here, Mr. T. Take this soapy cloth and wash as much as you can in the front. Do your privates, please."

Dad howled with joy when the shower was turned on full. The noise brought Mom to the door.

"What's happening? Is Bob all right?" she asked anxiously.

"Yes, Mother," I said soothingly. "We are leaning how to give Dad a shower. It's his first, and he loves it."

Minutes later, he stood at attention outside the shower stall, grabbing his trusty cane while Carrie rubbed him dry. She handed him the towel and he smudged his chest dry with loud "ho-ho-ho's" of pleasure and pain—pleasure that he could actually perform an activity by himself, and pain because part of his body was still unfeeling.

Taking a shower is quite an accomplishment on the road to recovery, and I am so grateful that I was here to watch an experienced nurse show us the technique to follow. I am sure that this will become part of his daily routine and I shall teach future aides, if they don't know the procedure.

TIME FOR MOM

October 3, 1978

Mother has her special times to sit with Dad, depending on her mood and the weather. Mornings she sits outside in the backyard. In the evenings she looks forward to reading a book aloud after dinner. Dad seems to understand, as he laughs and cries at the right places. Of course he cries easily, as most stroke patients do, for laughter and tears are very close.

The five o'clock cocktail hour is a must, and Mother and Dad always celebrate with a drink—rum and ginger ale for Mom, and plain ginger ale for Dad—unless she is too tired, too sick, or too involved in a book.

This job is so exhausting—getting Dad up and down many times a day, tying and untying his sling, buttoning up his sweater. We open and close doors, take him to the bathroom, do up zippers and belts, put Dad to bed, get him up, serve meals, take him to the beach and shopping, and do the household chores. No aide can work here more than three days at a time. That's why we stagger days and I work Sundays and Thursdays.

I go to the Nursing Home three days a week and work with Mom twice a week, which gives me two days off. The aide also gets two days off, working a full week with Dad.

Part of my problem has been that I did not know my job. When I ask aides for help, they often answer, "You're the Activity Director; why ask us?" I have been asking about previous activities, what other teachers did, etc. I've attended meetings with other activity directors and found that getting along with aides is often a problem as they have been taught to take orders only from nurses, and I hate to go through channels. I find it so easy to just ask, "Can you help me push so and so to the activity?" Sometimes they cooperate; sometimes they don't.

The result is that I am often grieved, upset and angry on the job as well as at home. I live in a world of older people and sick people. I've lost my former self. Oh, it's good experience, I suppose, but I find that I am often cursing or crying, and I am very tired every night. I am ill from exhaustion. My feet and hands curl up, and I have to go to bed at eight, leaving no time for my private life.

Something has to be done.

THE EST TRAINING

October 9, 1978

Today I learned that the EST Training is to be given in Miami. I'm thrilled because I thought that New York was the closest Center.

I heard Werner Erhard, founder of EST, speak in San Francisco in 1976. I didn't understand much of his speech, which had to do with "transforming your ability to experience living so that the situations you are trying to cope with, or put up with, clear up just in the process of life itself."

There was something magnetic and alive about the gathering of graduates, as if their eyes had been opened. A special electricity in the air warmed and united thousands of people as though we were all one family. I asked a young man beside me, "Have you done the training?"

"Yes."

"What did you get out of it?"

"I learned to take responsibility for my own life."

Jesus said it another way: "Take up your bed and walk." I know now that the training is something I want to do. I must explore my anger and learn who I really am. I want to see life more objectively, and learn to take responsibility, if possible.

Today I threatened my boss, half in jest, "You'd better be nice to me or I'll write about working here." She knows I took this job to find out what goes on behind the walls of a Nursing Home.

I signed up for the EST Training.

October 17, 1978

I came home after a weekend in the EST Training feeling like a heated coal.

During a "danger process," a large group of us stood on stage, staring into the audience. We had to learn to "be with" someone else and my eyes became riveted to a darkly bearded young man in the front row who reminded me of a Biblical character. He sent so much love from intense brown eyes that my spine began to tingle, and warmth spread through me. I felt like a terminal and was unable to give, only to receive the waves of power. Love, I thought, is electricity—we are all made up of vibrations.

During the two-day seminar, I had been dressed in a heavy coat, wool scarf, and ski cap, unable to get warm. Now I felt warm and free from pain. The glow seemed to last for several days. When I arrived at Bortz Monday morning after three hours sleep, I greeted my boss with a glowing smile. She looked at me stupefied, and exclaimed:

"Something's happened to you!" I grinned in response. Perhaps I had learned that when I felt afraid of others, they were actually afraid of me. We are mirrors of each other.

November 16, 1978

My life here at Bortz has changed as a result of my EST Training. I am able to "be with" my patients in a way that I never was before. I have learned the value of stooping so that I am at eye level with the seated or bedridden patients. It really makes a difference. I'm sure that they can feel how I care about them individually.

I have decided to stay on another year and I've set a goal of obtaining one hundred volunteers. (In the end, I stayed two years and obtained more than 200 volunteers).

December 5, 1978

I have broken a barrier at the local newspaper. When I originally suggested that they do stories about our work, they told me that "No one wants to read about old folks in nursing homes." Now they are beginning to do feature stories about us.

We have been inundated with children and church groups this month. People bring cookies and other gifts and sing for the patients, cheering them immensely.

My life at Bortz has also improved because I no longer insist on trying to do it my way. I have come to respect the aides and am going through channels, telling the head nurse when I need help. The aides are more willing to cooperate when the request doesn't come directly from me.

In dealing with the patients, I begin to see each as an individual with a unique set of needs and interests. I try to bring about truthful group sharing, as we did in the EST Training. That teaches each person to listen—and eventually opens up the space for them to become responsible for each other.

At home, I do not blow my cool as much, since I no longer feel that I am the "victim of circumstances." I have decided to attend an EST Seminar which gives me an opportunity for an additional mini-seminar, while driving with two other graduates to Miami. I guess you might call it my support system, which I so badly need.

In the seminar, we share our thoughts and feelings with a qualified leader who helps us look at our problem and take responsibility for it. When we do, we find that we have the capacity to make decisions on how to handle it. I can take what I learn to others. By sharing our lives and feelings, we are filled with power. We can begin to know, understand, forgive, and accept others and ourselves.

December 10, 1978

After the EST Training, I began to realize that I am actually responsible for everything that happens in my life. This extends even to what another person does, and so we are all responsible for the whole.

I asked myself: When does it stop being "them" who did it to me, and start being *my* responsibility? Am I willing to do what it takes to get things done? Is it always "them" or "they," "he" or "she," who created it a certain way, or is it my responsibility? My word makes it so.

MY COMMITMENT:

How I think it is, it is.

How I say it is, it is.

How I believe it is, it is.

I realize it's no use to fight being here with Mom and Dad, but that I chose to be here; and *if* I chose to be here, it's because I chose *not* to put Dad in a home. So after I recognize that it is, after all, my choice, I can no longer be angry with "them" for creating it this way. It just IS and I must accept it.

When I can recognize that this is it, this is the way things are, I can make a choice on how I want to deal with it.   I really feel some of my anger has dropped away and I am eager to share the EST experience with others.

December 17, 1978

Mom twisted her back a month ago and has been sleeping almost around the clock ever since. A vertebra in the lower back is pinching the sciatic nerve and she is in much pain and has trouble standing, walking or sitting.

I took her twice to a chiropractor who put blocks under her hips to straighten her back while he was working on her. She seemed better at the time but ended up in bed again. She has taken all kinds of pills for pain. Each new doctor prescribes something different. I have urged the aides to stop her from trying to help Dad stand or sit, lift the bed rails, or do the wash.

In October, she had a skin cancer on her face removed and she has had to wear a large hat when she goes outdoors. I do believe that Dad's persistent "Ha-ha-ha's" have worn her down. I was here only two days at a time and found it nerve-wracking

December 19, 1978

Dad has another urine infection, which is probably why

he's been yelling so much. It's difficult to know what's wrong with an aphasic. We have to be able to read his gestures.

We now have to keep a constant check on his urine, taking samples to the doctor. It's also a constant hassle to get his bowels to move. The aides make a daily report in the record book we have labeled "Mr. T." This keeps us in communication with each other. We note the medicine taken, daily exercise given, his mental and emotional state, meals, activities, and guests.

Today Mom got up for awhile. She tried to appear busy writing Christmas cards, but her memory is fading. Although she doesn't complain about the pain, she is now the one to be watched and nursed back to health. We are not keeping good track of the pills she has taken. It's hard enough caring for Dad.

Although Mom spends part of her time in bed reading, it's her sleeping that really frightens me. When a person in the nursing home becomes a bed patient, that is usually the beginning of the end, our doctor says. The heart function weakens and the blood doesn't circulate properly. We should take away all drugs but Ascription or Aspirin and locate the pain while she still remembers.

Don is coming and we are all restless in anticipation of his arrival.

December 20, 1978

Mom slept poorly and woke complaining of severe back pain. I took her to a doctor, who expressed confusion. Earlier, she had pain only when she was putting weight on her leg; now she's had two nights of pain while simply lying in bed. The doctor recommended an orthopedic surgeon.

December 22, 1978

Don had suggested that we consider putting both Mom and Dad in a nursing home and we checked on the costs. "They charge $28 a day for a semi-private room, excluding medication, doctors' care, laundry, hair-cutting, etc.," he wrote me. "They presently have sixty patients. They are accredited by the state, have RN's, LPN's and aides, according to state regulations. A doctor must see them monthly. Probably very perfunctory."

December 29, 1978

I wasn't feeling well this morning and Mom tried to get breakfast. She was lurching like a drunken sailor and her speech was slurred. She had been in a great deal of pain and I think she's taken too many pills. She had taken two Tylenol's at 4 a.m. and a Quaalude at 5 a.m. Now she wanted a Cortisone shot.

"No," I told her. "That's a bad habit. We have to find a doctor to fix your back." Her face was ashen and her hand bluish white. I nearly called an ambulance, but decided to lug her back to bed instead. She slept until noon.

January 2, 1979

I've been ill with the flu. When I recovered, I took Mom to another chiropractor, a huge powerful person who is God-led. Mom complained that he had hurt her, but I noticed that she walked when she got home.

January 10, 1979

Mom's back pain persists and I made an appointment with an orthopedic surgeon who X-rayed her, pointed to a suspicious area and said, "She could have cancer!" I was not convinced.

"Perhaps it's a broken rib from her last chiropractic treatment," I suggested, remembering how she had complained that he had hurt her.

"I don't think so," he replied.

January 15, 1979

After spending a week frightened silly, I learned that the suspicious area on the X-ray was NOT cancer, but a broken rib as I had suspected. I'm greatly relieved. The broken rib is a small price to pay for the good the wonderful doctor did her. He dared to give a seventy-nine-year-old woman chiropractic treatment for her sciatic nerve. I feel he saved her life as she had been sleeping so long that her health was severely endangered. She is walking again and has no further trouble with her leg.

February 4, 1979

I seemed to have attained an equilibrium between working with Dad and my job at Bortz, where I can serve the patients, working one on one, or in groups. I love the job. There are a number of people and groups to contact—volunteers, church groups, the college, newspapers, schools, etc. I have built up a pool of approximately two hundred volunteers who appear to gain more than they give.

We now offer the patients musicians, performers, travel films, ceramics, sewing, Bible study, news discussion, theater parties, picnics and Remotivation classes (which I enjoy teaching.) All these activities aid in bringing more stimulation and happiness to my larger Bortz family. There are many needs to be met and I have a feeling of accomplishment.

At home I still tangle with Mom and Dad. My experience at Bortz, however, has helped to validate my word and status. Our visits to Bortz have opened up new friendships for Dad and helped me to understand him better. Perhaps my experience with Dad has helped me understand my patients. It works both ways.

I still work at home as an aide two days a week, taking care of Dad as well as washing, cleaning, shopping and running the household. Mom and I continue to argue over what socks, shoes, pajamas, shirt or sweater Dad should wear. The final decision often rests with him as he indicates his choice with gestures. Other times, he seems to be saying, "What about me? Stop arguing, you two!"

He wants harmony.

March 10, 1979

Dad has definitely improved. Although they told us he would probably reach a plateau in six months, he reached a plateau, stayed there a year or so and moved on. I was surprised to hear myself dub him "Rugged Robert" in a course called "New Directions for Women" at Indian River Community College.

I have taken the course twice now, as it helped me through the first difficult year. I can relate to other women of all ages, unburden my emotions, and look at myself objectively. We had to give ourselves an adjective and I called myself "Dexterous Doris," as I am writer, painter, singer-dancer-actress, and now "aide" and activities director.

Dad is rugged, I thought, surprised to acknowledge that I admired this man. He is the same father whose domination and anger I resented in my youth, the same man who kept Mother on the end of a tether, and whose children were often petrified in his presence. He has demonstrated the power of persistence, which irritated us as children and now is saving his life. It takes persistence and courage to fight a stroke. Although these qualities come mainly from the patient, a lot depends upon the support of the family and their attitude towards his recuperation.

On looking back, I am proud of us all for the bull-headed tenacity with which we pressed on. We are grateful to God for the little accidents along the way, which led us to friendly people who contributed their time, effort and love.

DAD WALKS ALONE

March 17, 1979

An active person by nature, Dad now strolls around the

house and grounds two or three times daily ... alone, stopping under a palm tree for shade, observing his plants, flowers and trees and the brush pile that needs to be burned.

For two years we have accompanied him as he walks around the house, dressed in sweater, hat and arm sling. If it is chilly, we dress him in the old button-down, pink wool sweater, which stretches over the paralyzed arm, creating a bulge.

Once slim, he is now more prominent in the abdomen, just enough to have difficulty zipping up his pants. Although he hasn't learned to dress himself, he has at least begun to get up alone from his chair, which contains an extra pillow. He can walk to the bathroom alone and sit down, but then he bleats for us to help him up. He will also walk to the side door in the Florida room, open it and step down several inches to the stoop (which I covered with indoor-outdoor carpeting in case he falls), turn in place and close the door. He drags the heavy paralyzed leg encased in a brace slowly and painstakingly along.

If I hear a loud yell, I fear he has been bitten by a snake or fallen to the ground. Dashing out, I usually find that his leg brace has come loose and he is unable to continue until I refasten it. He's like a huge ship and I am the tiny tugboat that keeps him on course.

CATASTROPHE

July 1979

I have just brought Dad back from the hospital after treatment for a broken rib, and I'm mortified. I have been on duty alone while Mother went to a wedding in Houston for a few days, taking a much needed vacation after the demanding schedule involved in caring for a stroke patient.

Yesterday after lunch I lay in the sun for half an hour. Then, drowsy with sleep, I carried the lawn chair into the garage and lay down on the cot. Before dozing off, I remembered thinking that I shouldn't leave Dad's cane by his bed as he might try to get up without my help. I fell asleep without acting on the thought, however, and drifted into a dream, in which I heard him calling. I awoke with a start and rushed into his room. Dad was sprawled on the floor, bawling in pain and fear.

I managed to pull him up onto a low stool, from there to a hassock, and from there into bed to recover. His face and lips were pale. Sometime later I helped him out of bed with difficulty and walked him around the house. I was greatly relieved to discover that his knees were working and he hadn't broken a leg. I asked him if he wanted to go to the hospital but he shook his head no.

I read him several chapters from "Two on an Island", which we both enjoyed. After serving "cocktails," I prepared dinner. When we sat down, he demanded hot milk. I had planned hot tea.

"I'll get the milk after we eat a hot meal, Dad," I called from the kitchen. "I 'm getting your tea." He sat with his head down and would not eat. Was he angry? I brought him the tea and his head was still down. Was his face turning yellow?

"Dad, please lift up your head. I want to see your face. How do you feel?" He did not look up.

"Dad, are you in pain?" No answer.

"I think you had better lie down," I suggested. After a few mouthfuls, he finally pushed his chair away from the table. I helped him walk back to bed and he lay down fully clothed. Again I suggested he go to the hospital for a checkup, but he didn't want to go. He lay back. His voice was lighter. He used less oxygen. He could not talk as loudly as before. I left the doors open so I could hear him if he called. I phoned a nurse and described the situation.

"Take his pulse," she ordered. It was strong and steady. "Good," she assured me. "His heart is OK. Now, can he breathe deep?" I returned to ask him. He shook his head, no.

"His rib is fractured or broken," she reported. "But it won't heal any better in the hospital. "Give him a pain pill and a liquid," she advised, "and tell him to breathe deep breaths a half hour after the pain pill."

I called the doctor and he confirmed the nurse's recommendation. "Maybe we can have him X-rayed later. Keep him home and observe him. Keep him comfortable and give water or liquids."

Another nurse friend warned, "Don't let him dehydrate. Watch him for pneumonia." Another friend's son, a paramedic, came over to take his blood pressure because I was so worried. He suggested that I wrap Dad's chest in an Ace bandage, but I didn't have one.

Dad looks better. He gives a choking breath now and then, and talks in a weak, rasping voice only one-third normal strength. He doesn't seem to be getting enough air to yell loudly. I am growing more certain that he has a broken rib.

11 p.m. Things seem to be under control. I'll see if I can make him breathe deep and take some water. I'm sad this had to happen because Mother will feel guilty that she left for a vacation. It could have happened, however, when he was with her. All was well before this.

It now looks as if perhaps Mother was right about not wanting to teach him to get up by himself. But who knows? A nurse once told me that Mom had kept him back a whole year by not letting him progress on his own.

Well, I suppose this is the price we must pay for Dad's independence. Life moves on and we never know what we should have done. We can only do our best, and learn to accept. This morning we went to the hospital and the break was confirmed. Too bad! Now he and Mother will have to gain confidence in walking all over again. The doctor and nurse were right. He will heal on his own at home.

TRIP TO MAINE

August 5, 1979

Dad has agreed to go to Maine. Hooray! I guess he feels more secure now that he can walk alone. He knows he must rough it at the cottage, as we have no electricity and little heat, except for a small gas stove in the bathroom and a fireplace in the living room. His walking will be limited to the porch, as the grounds are uneven and full of roots.

I have two good aides who will care for Mom and Dad while I drive to Maine in the Chrysler. They will put my parents on the plane at West Palm Beach, and Don will meet them in Bangor. Don is urging me to take a vacation away from the folks but I really want to see my little brother, and I love being in Maine.

August 9, 1979

Driving north, I leave the Maine turnpike to take the rolling straight road to Belfast. The Maine air is invigorating and every hill brings a new perspective. New hope! I relish the picturesque farmhouses, the quaint white-spired churches set on grassy hillsides on the winding road to South Brooksville. Turning off the main road at the Norvega sign, I begin the two-mile drive through a wild stretch of woodlands leading to the water—and home.

A wrought-iron sign denotes our cottage, "Gull Rock," so named for a white gull which settles eloquently upon a large rock in front of our house every time the tide recedes. Dad loves the cottage, or at least he did after adding three picture windows, which lighten an otherwise dark interior.

From the couch in the living room, he can look out on a glorious view of Penobscot Bay with thirteen islands, green-jeweled in the sun. Little Deer Isle lies across Eggemoggin Reach. From our front porch, a short path leads through tall grass to the cragged rocks at the water's edge, where we lie in the sun or hold our yearly lobster cookout. The rocks form a "bathtub" where children can play and from which we venture into the cold blue waters to glide through swaying seaweed as we look down at the clear rocky bottom.

The dining room faces a sharp cliff of rocks edged with clumps of evergreen trees, which line the road leading to the cove. Here we keep three boats—a dingy, a motorboat and a sailboat, "Fledgling." She is the reason our men folks love Maine. Although I like to sail, I almost prefer to be in the water or standing at a wooden table under the pines, where I used to sculpt heads out of granite. The rock was my guru, as I had to make many drawings to be able to see three-dimensionally. Every blow of hammer and chisel took energy, precision and thought.

Our rustic two-story cottage includes a kitchen, a tiny downstairs bedroom (where Dad will sleep), and a bathroom. Running water from a well allows us to live in luxury, warming up after a cold swim with a small trickle of water from a makeshift shower.

At night we read by gaslight and retire upstairs with a flashlight to one of four small bedrooms whose unique feature has always been a source of embarrassment to me. The dividing walls don't reach the slanted roof and night sounds are magnified. We can hear anyone turning over, snoring, using a potty or descending creaky stairs to visit the bathroom or rob the refrigerator. I prefer sleeping on the studio couch in the living room where I can look out the window and watch the dawn paint the sky pink, sometimes meditating on a rock at the magic time before the wind ruffles the glass-like bay.

Arriving at the cottage at 8 a.m., I find that Don has organized a routine and is bathing Dad in the bathroom, the only warm room in the house. Before breakfast, we must start the pump, replenish the woodpile, gather kindling and make a fire in the fireplace.

Dad cried when he saw me and Hi-Tail. Was it because I had arrived safely, or because he had finally made it to Maine? Actually we both made it, and I am quite proud.

August 12, 1979

Today I watched Dad walk back and forth across the porch.

"Twenty times, Dad," Don urged. "You've only done ten so far." I believe Dad can count. Don exercises him faithfully every morning and is determined to play the male nurse, giving Mom and me a break. My writing is spread upon the dining room table until dinnertime.

At noon, Don evaluates the weather for sailing. If the waters are choppy and the winds brisk, it could be a good day for sailing. If the waves dash against the rocks, churning into a foamy white spray, the water is dangerous. When squalid eccentric gusts create cross-hatches of rippling waves, we can expect to become becalmed or tossed about in an angry sea.

Due to his illness the last three years, Dad had been unable to come to Maine for the first time in sixty years. As Don says, he was unable to accept his infirmity, vacillating between rage and despair. He was rudderless, beached, and no longer able to answer the call of the wind and the sea.

SAILOR

Earthbound, his ship is scuttled now;

Broken the hull, damaged the prow,

Paralysis has maimed the bow.

His grip, that once held sheeting fast,

Has loosed its hold—broken, the mast;

'Twas life's surrender, mournful task.

Dad was a fine sailor who kept his boat shipshape, demanding perfection from a sluggish crew. Now his lungs can no longer expand with the gale, his arms can no longer let out the sail in a reach. He is harbored, docked. Our family wallows in his "Wa-wa-wa's." Sometimes he rails so loudly and with such urgency that if I am in another part of the house I run quickly into the living room sure that he has fallen, only to find him pointing excitedly to a passing schooner under full sail. A tiny sailboat receives the same cries of happiness. He is like a small boy with his first toy. We share his joys as well as his agony that he will never sail again.

Our little town of South Brooksville consists of a Congregational Church, a grocery store, a post office and the Bucks Harbor Yacht Club. Dad was commodore for half a season and ran the Saturday races. There are two races a week and often the fleet sails by our cottage. Members congregate for the awards at Saturday teas.

On Thursday evenings, our family often piles into the car to attend square dances at the club. Over the years, we have watched children grow up, get married and return with tots of their own. To many of us summer people, Maine is our only "roots," as our jobs take us from town to town and state to state.

Our family has visited South Brooksville for twenty-five years. Mother has summered in Sedgwick, only seven miles away, since she was six years old. Her grandfather, Charles Nelson Rhodes, owned the old Carlton House, a stately mansion overlooking the Benjamin River.

My childhood includes many pleasant memories of hay rides, picnics in the pine grove, eating outdoors under a huge tree, swinging in the hammock, clamming at low tide and swimming in the cove with cousins and relatives.

Dad has returned to Norvega, to his summer roots and the land he loves so well. Like the seagull returning to Gull Rock, he has come home again. Although we may have thought that he strayed from his course, giving in to the cruel demands of stroke, I realize that he was only on a tack, headed for his goal.

"But Dad, why can't we go right towards our destination," I asked as a young girl, when Dad took me sailing. "Why do we have to travel all around it and not even aim for it?" The mystery of the wind and sail and the techniques of sailing were beyond me then as they are now.

He explained in his taciturn manner, "Choose a goal and stick to it! Then set your sail so you don't luff. It's like the game of life. Do that and you'll get there. Sometimes the weather will make you change your direction, but never give up on your goal."

And Dad never has. As a stroke patient in Jensen Beach, he faithfully exercised every day so he could walk again. He walked so he could return to Maine. Despite the depression, frustration and anger, he accomplished his goal by forging windward against the wiles of stroke.

If it were not for Dad's perseverance and dogged determination, he would never have improved enough to make this trip, fulfilling his deepest desire. He loves the surly, primitive mountains, the land of sudden-thickening fog that blots out the sun and holds you captive for two hours, two days, or two weeks, until finally the yellow blur melts through the milky white day to reveal a shiningly beautiful blue and green world.

Tonight after supper, Dad made a few more tacks on the porch, then settled back in his red rocking chair to watch every magnificent nuance of the glowing sunset, groaning with gentle "Ah's" over the lavender, red, and orange designs mirrored in the glittering waters of the bay.

PART FIVE

ACCEPTANCE

(May 13, 1980 – February 1981)

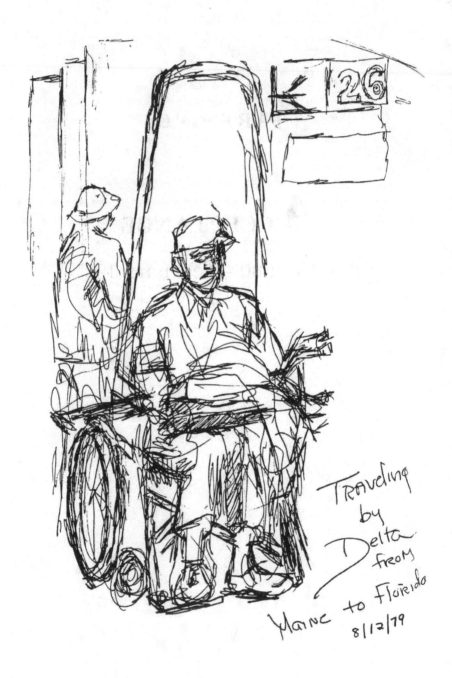

26

Traveling
by
Delta from
Maine to Florida
8/17/79

V

TURNING POINT

May 13, 1980

This has been a heavy day. I must accept the fact that Mom's mind is deteriorating. Now our roles are reversed. The mother I'd always counted on to take care of me now needs my care. I suppose this had to happen eventually, as the pressure on her has been so great.

It started when I returned from a vacation in Nassau. When I'd taken off, I had been sure that I'd left my parents in competent hands. We had hired an aide named Carol, a lithe, flashy blonde. Divorced with two young children, she lived with her mother. I thought that she was a bit overly sugary with Dad, but he basked in her attention. She had been taking him to the beach, which both of them seemed to enjoy—she, undoubtedly because the boys swarmed around her like honey.

My first doubts came when I returned to a filthy house. Then I discovered that five pages had been torn out of the calendar. This upset me because I had been recording Carol's hours on the calendar and now had an incomplete record. She hadn't yet asked me for any of her pay, but I had assumed that was because she was living with her mother and didn't need the money yet. I thought she might want her money in one big payment.

But when I upbraided her about tearing out the pages, she denied it and then mentioned casually that the hours didn't matter because Mother had been paying "us" all along.

I was stunned. Carol and I had reached agreement on three points before she was hired. We had settled the amount of her paycheck, that I would pay her, and that Mother was not to write a check. The week she got the job, she asked Mother for more money. I said no. Now I realized too late that Mother had been writing checks behind my back.

"Us?" I asked sharply.

"Oh, my mother came a few times to do some hard cleaning. She did the windows and cleaned the house," Carol said blithely.

When I found Mother's checkbook, I was stunned. Mom had been paying these two women a total of $400 a week for several weeks. What a fool I had been. This will be the third time I shall have to fire women for going "over my head," so to speak. The worst part of it is that I am fighting Mother at the same time I am fighting the aides. And I have Dad fighting me! I am sorry to do this to Dad. Both women really liked him. Or so it appeared. I guess they liked the money, too.

There must be a solution. I cannot live like this much longer. I called the Health and Rehabilitation Services and a woman will come tomorrow, a social worker.

SOCIAL WORKER

May 14, 1980

The social worker came today, a competent woman in her thirties. She and Mom sat on the front porch and chatted amicably.

I explained the situation and wanted to see if she would detect Mother's senility, as I needed some guidance and support as to what to do next. Mother answered her questions correctly, but talked mostly of the past. There was no way for the woman to know that Mom is unable to handle daily routines. She doesn't know what day it is, how to write a check correctly, or how to take and give messages correctly over the phone.

The woman decided that Mom is fine and I am still up a tree. If only Mother would realize that I am on her side and fighting for her. But no! She still wants to act the autocratic ruler, albeit a forgetful one.

In desperation, I went to the doctor with my problem. He wrote me a report about Mother's senility. I guess he has seen it all along. Stress because of Dad's stroke (and with me, perhaps), has brought on deterioration of her body, as well as her mind. I am helpless to do anything, however, unless I can be strong enough to hurt her. I know she will never understand.

"Mother," I began today, trying to explain. "We have arranged for the girls to be paid through the Trust Officer who takes care of Dad's affairs. I am to send in the hours they worked. You were paying them and not telling me. We can't live like this with two bosses. Every girl I hire asks you for a raise, and you give it to her. $400 a week is a preposterous amount of money to pay—even for 'hard cleaning.' It was hard all right, on us!"

"Doris, I'm still the boss here and I'll pay people if I wish. It's my money!" Her eyes flashed.

"But it's my life! And I'm not going to waste it by fighting you and watching your money and your lives go down the drain, and be unable to do anything about it. If you want to run this house, then I'll have to leave, because it's not working this way."

"So leave. Go back to your house and stay there," she spat. The poor woman! She does not seem to realize that I have been running the whole show here for years, or trying to.

"Mother, I can't live like this in two places. I lug my heavy electric typewriter back and forth between two houses, my books, my shoes, my clothes, my cat. I'm living out of my truck and I have trouble getting dressed because I don't know where my bra is."

I pleaded, cajoled, begged and finally threatened. "We've got to do something. We'll have to put Dad into a nursing home or take away your checkbook. After all, you're paying the Trust Officer to pay the bills and yet you continue to pay them. And you can't even remember to write on the stubs the amount you have spent and to whom!"

It's like trying to save a drowning woman who is pulling you under. What shall I do? Sometimes I hate her. And I know she hates me. I guess she wants it like it used to be, as Dad used to be. But it's different. I've spent four years of my life helping them. Perhaps I wasn't too successful before, but I'm certainly not successful now.

I spoke to the Trust Officer today. He suggested I hide her checkbooks, hoping she won't notice. Oh, God, if only she could realize that I'm on her side. I've fired the women and it's depressing around here.

JUGGLING ACT

May 17, 1980

I called my brother, Bob, to tell him what is happening and he bawled me out. Carol had already called him and complained. The audacity of some people! So now I even have my family against me.

I can't imagine why Bob would listen to her and not to his own sister. I tried to explain, and told him what I intended to do. Today Mother asked for her checkbook and I suggested very kindly that she let me take care of the money and bills from now on.

"What shall I do if I can't write a check?" she wailed. "I would feel worthless. I'm not even a person. I might as well be dead."

And I am dying! My brother can't understand why we should cancel Mother's check book and I don't have the heart to do it. We are already sending the bills to the trust officer and I am buying the groceries.

Watching Mother's fear, I now understand what an older person goes through when deprived of the ability to write checks. I understand why some of the ladies at the Nursing Home continue to carry around their pocketbooks even though there is no money in them. They are used to being independent and find it hard to accept the change. Somehow, writing a check identifies you as a person. You can write your own ticket, call the shots. But to lose that right is like becoming a child again. Taking away the checkbook denies one the right to make decisions. That is what this is all about. Power! One's future is in jeopardy when one can't pay one's way.

I think of a patient at Bortz, who only yesterday had looked at me in helpless confusion.

"I have no money to pay for this hotel room tonight. Where am I going to sleep? Can you help me?" she asked pitifully.

"Now don't worry. It's all been taken care of. You can stay here as long as you want to. You're not to worry about money," I counseled. "You took care of your family all of your life, and now they're taking care of you." How to know what to say? She'll remember this for a few minutes and then she will ask again.

Speaking of money, I am now being paid for my two days aide service, because I went through all of my savings while making myself available for Mother. I was unable to take a steady job, as I had to alternate with the aides. And I didn't want to be away from here, because I am really the one responsible for the decisions about Dad's exercise, etc. And obviously I must keep an eye on the aides, as well as on Mother. It's been a juggling act. I am balancing Mom, Dad and the aides. And half of the time, I am also up in the air.

When I share my problems with the head nurse at Bortz, she urges me to put Dad in a home. She says I will not be able to live through it and seems to think my life is in danger.

It looks as if all communication has broken down now, mostly because there are no clear lines of responsibility in this murky undertow. I pray to find a way out.

JOINT CHECKING ACCOUNT

May 18, 1980

We are to have a joint checking account. I will do the shopping as usual. In fact, I have been doing everything again. I had to leave my job at the home. They needed a full-time activity director, as a new extension will soon be completed and there will be an additional sixty patients in the new wing.

I am just as happy, as the job was killing me physically. My hands were swollen and painful and would not straighten out. My feet hurt; I had trouble breathing and had high blood pressure several times. On one occasion, for example, I walked down the hall like a tilting ship. Aides took my blood pressure and found it very high and made me lie down in a reclining chair with my feet higher than my heart for hours.

Well, I have moved most of my clothes to a bureau in the garage and will sleep on the cot, or in the living room. I must get a new aide soon as working twelve hour shifts with Dad is difficult for any one person.

MISHAP

May 20, 1980

Dad has fallen several times in the house. Once, when he tried to get up and straighten the books on my side table; another time when coming in the front door with Mother. For some reason, they both lost their balance walking up the ramp, and went down together on the living room rug. Thank God nobody was hurt.

Today, however, I heard a howl on the lawn outside Mother's bedroom window and rushed out. I found Dad sprawled on the grass yelling in pain and terror. He had tripped over a garden hose left in his path by the man who cuts the lawn once a month.

Although frightened, I tried to remain calm and helped him to sit up. I knew I couldn't stand him up alone.

"Sit here, Dad, and don't move. I'm going for help and I'll bring a stool." I ran next door and shouted for Ursula.

"What's wrong?" She appeared at the door, two Doberman Pinschers at her side. Heavy-set, likable and German, she was the only friend within shouting distance.

I explained and dashed to the garage to find a low stool. We returned to Dad who was still helpless, stunned and crying.

"So you've taken a fall, Bob? No problem," Ursula said soothingly.

"Please God," I prayed silently. "Let him be all right."

I placed the stool behind him and together we helped him to sit. From there it was another lunge to lift him into a standing position. I walked him back into the house and put him to bed.

He is still crying and I wonder if he broke anything. He doesn't want to go to the hospital, but I'll find out eventually.

LEILA ANN

May 24, 1980

I discovered my friend, Leila Ann, on the beach today. She was barefoot and wearing a nurses outfit. A large-boned young woman in her early twenties, she is tall and extremely attractive with a Franz Hal's kind of beauty. Her skin is like that of a ripe peach.

When she came to my door requesting art lessons several years ago, I had been disconcerted by this oversized woman and felt diminutive in her presence. Beneath her astonishing exterior, however, I discovered a little girl soul.

"Leila Anne! What are you doing here and where have you been," I exclaimed.

"I went home to Ohio for six months, but I got bored and came back," she said. "And I need a job desperately," she added.

"But why the uniform? Have you been working?"

"I bought the uniform for twenty-five cents at a thrift shop," she admitted with a disarming smile, and then added, "but I have worked as a Nurses Aide. I love working with old people."

I felt God was painting the picture, answering my prayers in the form of Leila Ann, for I had made my needs known this morning before going swimming.

"Well, we need someone at Mother's house in Jensen as my father had a stroke four years ago. How would you like to come home with me right now and look the situation over?" She agreed and we tumbled into the van, wet bathing suit, nurse's outfit and all.

May 25, 1980

Mother and I have been at each other's throats again. Sometimes I think all her "Dearie, sweetie-pie sweet talk" to Dad is really pity for herself. We've all been in anguish since I fired the two women. I've been sick with laryngitis and several times a day I've had to string Mom's head up in traction as her neck hurts. We'd been struggling along by ourselves until yesterday when Leila Ann appeared.

Leila Ann and I now spell each other. Thanks to her experience in nursing homes, she realized that Dad has an infection. He has been listless, has baggy eyes, and has been pointing to his stomach in pain. He is now taking medicine. Lethargic, he does not want to don cap and sweater or take his morning walk ever since he fell over the hose.

He did not break anything, thank God.

ON LEAVING BORTZ

May 27, 1980

Having decided to leave Bortz Spring Lake, I realize that I shall miss the patients immensely. It is like leaving a dear family I have come to love. Trying to put my feelings into words tonight, I wrote the following letter to my successor:

Letter To a New Activity Director:

I bequeath to you the many faces of Eve you will encounter. And Adam, in all his wilting splendor.

I bequeath courage to the frail sparse frame of a ninety-two year-old woman who lies curled up on her bed like a dried leaf, holding tightly to your fingers as she clings to life, saying, "I'm ready to go. Hold my hand. Don't leave me!" Her eyes blaze with aliveness above the impish grin. Yesterday she played ball and bingo, her mind bright as a new copper penny. You want to stay with her—just to be there.

I bequeath to you the many wheelchairs you must push several times a day, the publicity you should write, the phone calls that don't get made, the unexpected joy of new volunteers whom God sends to you just when you need them most.

I bequeath to you the joy you feel on a lazy May morning while listening to born-again Christians talking of Jesus; the search for truth in the Good Book; and the blind lady's hasty answer, which is always so perfect—as though she can see better than the rest of us with eyes; and her impatience when we don't "get on with it."

I bequeath to you the gem of them all, blind Woody, who never gets enough "real" people to read to him. Sitting in his rocker every night between 6 and 8 p.m., he wishes for some human being to come and chat, to read from Guideposts, to discuss the news, share old times or ask important things of life, like: "Why am I still here at eight-five, blind and healthy? God must have a job for me to do. Am I doing it?"

Yes, Woody. You hold us together with your strength, your willingness and eager cooperation, your gentlemanly bearing, your positive, cheerful attitude, your grace and humility.

I bequeath to you the many groups of church ladies who will come to help, to preach, to sing, to serve cookies and just to be a friend.

I bequeath to you miles of new hallways, white walls and

colored doorframes. And new faces of Eve—a senior citizen with blurred eyes who answers: "My children? Oh, one's in Jacksonville ... maybe Detroit. They can't come down. They're busy."

And the boat trips! The smiling faces at picnics and plays; quiet times on the porch alone with memories; a crow on top of a telephone pole; and all the hammering, plastering and electrical wiring you missed while we were pregnant with birth pains of our new building.

I bequeath to you the staff of dedicated people who have worked here as aides in the food service department, as nurses, doctors or housekeepers.

And most of all, I bequeath to you the care-ridden faces of those families who must bring their loved ones here. What more can some of us do when faced with the insurmountable difficulties of senility—the endangered species! These are the smiling nonsensical wise ones whose words become atrociously entangled, but you know the thought behind the mangled phrase. You nod with them and understand.

I bequeath to you the laughter, the tears, the heartache— the loved ones you must part with, those you'll grow fond of. The retarded, the whisperer, the glarer, the singer, the bookworm, the loner, the busy-body; the TV watchers and the bitter self-destructive ones. And the blind, who learn each day the meaning of the words, "Wait on the Lord. Wait, I say, and I shall give you PEACE."

Ah, life is a continual open door. When one door shuts, another opens. I bequeath to you the springtime of your life. For isn't GIVING always springtime, no matter what one's age? And isn't learning a continual experience? Accept what you can do. Accept what IS and go beyond yourself. I did.

But now I need a rest and I bequeath to you my job. Let me step aside awhile and look at Life, while you must gaze on Death. Life is a continual parting and becoming.

I bequeath to you days of mixed amends and incompletions. Just your smile, your style, your love. These are important.

Until we meet again,

An Activity Director

P.S. I must rest awhile, rest my body, my throat, my mind. I must take time to polish up my dreams I must look into the mirror and see who I really am before I am ready to go . . . Oh, my people—I love you so.

INVITATION

June 3, 1980

Robert's son, "Jeffy-Boo" is scheduled to marry in June. I remember him as a baby when, in an effort to sketch his portrait, I had to barricade myself behind tables and chairs. Now a young lady named Lynn has caught him and we are invited to the wedding in Houston. Jeff is studying to be a pediatrician.

"I want to take Dad," Mother announced eagerly. "We wouldn't miss it for the world." Truly, it would be an occasion, as neither Don nor I had married. My brother Bob's oldest son, Scott, also a doctor, had married an anesthesiologist, and it doesn't look as if a baby is in the ether because they are both in love with their work. Our only hope for an extension of the family line lies in Jeffy-Boo and his wife to be.

The idea of Dad flying to Texas, however, is out of the question. How could we be sure that Dad would not pull a tantrum in a public place? The only solution, I feel, would be for Mother or me to go alone—or together.

"Mother," I remonstrated. "How can you expect to fly Dad to Texas when you won't even let me drive him to Palm Beach to visit the Rehabilitation Center?" The airport is in West Palm Beach.

"We're going," she retorted. "It's final."

"But Mother," I protested. "Suppose we get all packed and ready to go and Dad won't budge? We'll have to stay home."

"Not another word. We'll all fly to the wedding."

"But Mother!" I felt like a dog with a meatless bone. "Suppose Dad howls at the wedding like he does sometimes in church? Robert would be horrified!"

"It's final."

The decision was hers. What could I do but go along with her and take our chances that Dad would cooperate. I called Bob with the news.

"Doris, are you crazy?" His voice mounted in anger. "Don't let Mother do it! There will be a big reception after the wedding and I will not have Dad imposed upon my guests."

"We're coming," Mother said calmly from the bedroom. I decided to let the situation resolve itself.

SHOPPING ESCAPADE

June 7, 1980

"Dad needs a new suit, I'm afraid. He's outgrown all of his pants and there is no suitable jacket for the wedding," Mother said today after breakfast. I was exercising Dad's leg.

"Push, Dad. Push! Push!" The leg was getting stronger.

Seated on the side of the bed, I held his weak foot against my shoulder and ordered him to push against me. "Good, Dad. You are improving. Now, how would you like to drive down town with me this afternoon and look for some clothes for the wedding?" He nodded his head yes, and I was thrilled. Perhaps we shall go to Texas after all!

I begged Mother to come with us shopping.

"No, dear, you two run along. Whatever you pick out will be fine." My heart fell. I knew nothing about men's clothes and was not at all sure that I could select an appropriate suit. I completely forgot about Dad's decisive mind, however.

Life is a cycle, I thought, as I guided Dad into a swanky men's store; he used to buy clothes for me and now I must buy for him. Suddenly I am the parent and he the child. A portly, silver-haired gentleman glided elegantly towards us.

"Sir, would you please help me dress my father for a wedding?" I asked. "I mean, I know nothing about men's clothes and ..." I blushed. He smiled and I led Dad to an easy chair. When I returned, the salesman gestured with a flourish and I gasped at the beautiful outfit displayed on a counter—natty pink and white checkered jacket, wine pants, and a dusky pink shirt topped by a creamy bow tie.

"Dad, come and see!" I exclaimed, visualizing how handsome he would look in this ensemble. After some delighted "Wa-wa-wa's," he approved of the selection and motioned for the salesman to wrap it up.

A French seamstress was called and Dad was invited to follow her to the dressing room. He balked, railing loudly. He would not be moved, and the distraught woman had to measure his leg as he stood at the checkout desk.

"Do you have something for him to travel in? Something bright?" I asked. Something eye-catching might prod our relatives into acceptance, helping to set the mood for a celebration. Within seconds, the salesman had scooped up a pair of fire-hydrant red pants, a suave navy and white checked jacket, and a string tie with the initial "R."

Dad was still wailing. His old impatience while shopping, even when it was for him, was still intact. He wanted to go home now, clothes or no clothes, wedding or no wedding. When he saw the bold red pants, however, he let out a surprised "Oh-oh-oh, ah!" followed by a gasping chortle. I paid the bill, escorted him to the car with two large boxes under one arm and a pleased feeling of accomplishment. Texas, here we come, ready or not.

That night I called Bob. "It looks like we're coming, Robert," I warned, not telling him about our purchases. "We've got our flight tickets."

"I hope you know what you're doing," he grumbled.

I crossed my fingers and waited. When the wine wedding

pants arrived, they were two inches too short, but it was too late to recoup.

TRIP TO TEXAS

June 13, 1980

Friday morning arrived. I was so nervous I forgot how to put on Dad's blue plaid jacket. Mother helped me. Of course, you put in the paralyzed arm first so he can bend the good arm. He looked wildly handsome and his excitement matched the occasion. When he finally walked obediently to the car, I heaved a sigh of relief.

How great to leave behind the house and all its anguish! We look forward to new sights, new people, new experiences. We can forget past grievances, the fear and anger. Dad and I sang lustily all the way to the station: "Old Mac Donald Had A Farm," "Easter Bonnet," "Bicycle Built for Two," etc. Dad was happy and he loves to sing. As he put nonsensical sounds to the old familiar tunes, I joined in with a kind of gibberish. We were like three school kids on a holiday. Dad, sitting beside me in the front seat, noted every new building with interest, howling in protest at broken ground.

A man met us at the airport with a wheelchair. Many "Wa-wa-wa's" later we were seated in the non-smoking section. Our exhilaration was contagious. There is something child-like about a stroke patient, as if he is seeing the world for the first time. Dad's curiosity and ability to absorb everything he sees is definitely an improvement over last year when his head drooped a lot. Now he holds his head up and looks much more normal, except, of course, when his face contorts into a tragic mask and the tears flow.

I am thrilled to be going back to Houston. I remember visiting as a little girl when we lived in Port Neches opposite an oil field. I was six, Bob was four, and Don was born there. Dad worked for the Texas Company, which he continued to do for the rest of his working life. I walked to school barefoot with a boyfriend who carried my books. A highlight of those years was when an elegant ship's Captain invited us on board his boat, set me on his lap and offered me sugar lumps. It was hard to believe that these succulent squares evolved from the sweet stalks, which grew in the field beside our house.

This trip is a little like sugar cane. It will be sweet, I hope, and surprising.

THE WEDDING

June 14, 1980

Dad behaved well at the wedding, crying only once. Standing transfixed at the rear of the church, he watched the diminutive brunette walking down the aisle dressed in a white ruffled hoop skirt with a twenty-foot-long lace train. His chest swelled with pride and his eyes glowed, wondering, perhaps, if this beautiful creature could really be his new granddaughter. What memories brought tears to his eyes? Was he thinking of his and Mom's wedding in Harvard Church, Brookline, Mass.?

We drove to the Doctor's Club at Baylor Medical School for the reception to be held in a huge ballroom. I was prepared for the worst. Would Dad be difficult and want to leave? How would he accept the noise and confusion? Would the cane and brace add to his embarrassment of being different?

We entered the crowded room. Three hundred people were gossiping, eating and drinking. We sat Dad at a side table and several people came over to congratulate him. He beamed, radiant in his new wine and pink outfit. Attending this event was a real triumph after all of our trials over the past four years. The sleepless nights listening for his moans; the anger over who would dress him and how; the arguments over whether or not we should take him to church; the moments of fear when we wondered whether he would live through the next day.

Dad nodded agreeably to folks who stopped by to say

hello. He did not whimper or howl. He wore his old social graces—and the pink jacket, over which he sported a new pink terry cloth bib edged with white bric-a-brac, one of three I had hastily sewn before our departure.

"Pop, you're the hit of the party!" Bob sidled up with a large grin. "Thank you for coming." This was worth our pain, effort and dilemma about coming. We had made it, thanks to Mom's courageous insistence.

I suggested we have a family picture taken to commemorate the event. Mom and Dad, Bob and his wife, Phyl, Jeff and Lynn, posed together happily. I was left out of the picture and that hurt a bit. But then, I could at least keep the picture.

That evening after a successful dinner party at which Dad was the star, I stopped to have a drink with Don under a Texas sky. The night was black as silk and Don's face glowed with a newly acquired tan, set off by a white dinner jacket. The beauty of the day was spoiled, however, when my brother suddenly began berating me.

"Doris, you are a total failure. Why are you wasting your life taking care of Dad? You are throwing your life away. They have lived their lives. Don't you think you deserve to live yours? I would never do what you are doing. I could never be expected to leave my teaching job and my students to spend my life taking care of a sick parent."

I was shocked. What should have been a celebration turned into a fiasco. I thought I had done a good job. I expected praise rather than accusations.

"But Don, you're not me." I groped for words to express myself. "It's a service. As I serve, I learn and grow. I've never had children and I've never had to care for anyone except when I taught occupational therapy in army hospitals."

Tonight was a milestone in Dad's rehabilitation. I felt proud of myself for this accomplishment, but Don could only see Dad's illness and my wasted life.

"Besides, I like it," I said. "I now know what it's going to be like to get old and infirm, to face death sometime in the future. I'm forced to deal with all the hate and rejection in the past, too. And my parents are somehow the first children I've had. Perhaps I'm also paying back a debt. Dad bought me the house in Stuart and I promised to contribute half towards the mortgage, but I never kept my word. Dad helped me when I was destitute. Now he needs my help. What else is there to do with my life?"

"But look at yourself, Doris. You're not a great actress and you always wanted to be. You're not a successful artist, and you're a good one. You're not even a writer. What are you? What are you doing with your life?"

Suddenly I felt as if I could see inside him, see his anguish. "Don," I agreed calmly, observing the pain in his eyes. "You're right. I can see that you are very upset and angry because I am a total failure."

He withdrew, slightly shocked. I had not followed my usual pattern of defense—tears and a cry for help.

"Well," he recapitulated. "You are not a total failure. After all, it was due to you and your activities in New York that I was led to art, dance and drama. I performed in dance and theater, visited art museums and plays. All these creative fields have affected my life and now I am teaching Chinese art. I am aware of the arts and you did it for me."

It was my turn to be astounded. I had not expected any compliments. I had merely looked upon his suffering as my own. I had, as we say in EST, recreated him. A moment ago, stripped of all pride, sense of accomplishment and self worth, stripped of all direction and receiving no acknowledgment for a job well done, I had looked back over the four years of frustration, anger and anguish endured with my parents, taking Dad's pain as my own. I was often at the end of my rope, not knowing which way to turn. Yes, I had given up my own life, my own goals in an effort to care for my father—helping to alleviate sickness, boredom, pain and frustration.

What was my brother trying to tell me? Could it be that he really believed in me? Was he trying in his own way to save my life, just as I had tried to save Dad's? What strange ways we humans choose to show love.

"Well, Don, I believe that I am stronger. Two years ago if you had spoken to me like that, I would have disintegrated in tears. But because I have taken the EST Training and continued to take seminars, I realize that I am responsible for what I choose to have in my life. And I don't choose it to be any other way right now. Thank you for caring."

He leaned back in his chair, looking at me thoughtfully.

"Perhaps you have changed for the best," he said gently.

We parted friends and went our separate ways.

WALKING THE TIGHTROPE

July 25, 1980

I am in Maine with my parents and Don. I traveled north on a bus after attending a writing Seminar in Atlanta and arrived at Norvega in the evening to find Dad seated in the dim dining room, a tray pulled close to his waist. His face contorted in tears when I kissed him hello.

All evening Dad's bleating "Ah's" and perpetual wails have battered my tired nerves. I am so utterly exhausted that every sound is magnified. I crave silence. I had forgotten this total disruption of the atmosphere. It's like having a baby to care for, as Dad must be attended to continually. But this baby won't grow up. Have Mom and I really put up with this for four years?

August 12, 1980

Life is a tightrope. You take another step and hope you make the right move and don't fall into the brink. I came here to be with my brother and because I love Maine. But I feel isolated, rejected and useless.

Don hired "Candy" full time with orders not to let Mother or me lift a finger. My God! Is this how Mother felt when the aides and I cared for Dad, rejecting her help, and ignoring her orders? Again the mountains shall be leveled. I feel good for nothing.

I take my work upstairs, type in the dining room or go outdoors to write. But I withdraw from Don, Candy and Dad, because they seem to have a special rapport that excludes me. Candy is sunny, a stocky ebullient Maine woman whom Don hired because he liked her spunk. He thought she could handle Dad, and they do get along fine.

Candy bathes and dresses Dad before breakfast. Don gets breakfast and Candy cooks lunch and dinner. Mom and I float around on the periphery, feeling exceedingly lost and useless even though Don, no doubt, meant to give us a vacation.

It is somehow cruel.

August 26, 1980

I am heartbroken over my brother's attitude towards me this summer. My "little" brother has always been the one family member I thought I could count on to support, understand and believe in me. He is the only one with whom I was "OK," regardless of my faults, idiosyncrasies, and my so-called failure to become socially or artistically successful.

But this summer he has completely changed his personality. His attitude towards me is different and I feel like a stranger, for he has become hard, unloving and cryptic.

Possibly it has to do with his friend who is visiting us, as there is no love lost between us. When he and his friend left the cottage, I felt a heavy weight lift from my shoulders. I could sing and laugh again. Candy was surprised that I am not the ogre Don painted me as being, and we have become good friends.

RAZOR EPISODE

Sept. 26, 1980

We are back in Jensen. Last night Dad roared at Mother for so long that I got up to help her. She had completed getting

him ready for bed and now sat beside him, unable to understand what he wanted.

"I'm tired. It's the end of the day and I want to get this
over with."

Dad understood, and wailed, apparently wounded at her
admission of weakness and fatigue.

Mother stood up, crumpled and unnerved. "What does he
want? I can't figure it out."

He pointed to the electric razor, which she had un-
plugged.

"He wants this plugged in," I said.

"But it's been in all day. He couldn't want it in again."

Dad's protests increased in volume and I plugged the razor in. He quieted.

"But it shouldn't be in that long," Mother said and she
started to unplug it. Dad began raving again and held up two
fingers, as if to refute her.

"Perhaps he means twenty-four hours," I suggested.
"Mother, Dad knows what he wants," I placated. "We shouldn't
argue with him. Now if only he would shave himself!" I placed
the electric razor in his hands, but to no avail.

This constant stress is wearing her down. Her face is becoming etched with strain, her back more stooped and bent.
Yet when she reads to him in their private moments, her face
is alive with drama.

So far we have read him "Heidi," which we all loved, "The
Little Princess," "Little Women" and "Little Men." We are grateful that his attention span has improved and that we have
found books to hold his interest.

ANOTHER GIRL FIRED!

September 1980

I have rehired Leila Ann and it's not working out. For one
thing, her housework is slipshod. For another, we don't seem
to be getting along the way we used to. Perhaps the fact that

I'm her "boss" is making it difficult for her to relate to me as a friend.

She has told me that she can't seem to hold a job longer than three months, and I told her that perhaps she is unconsciously trying to force me to fire her. I asked her if she wanted to try an EST exercise with me. When she agreed, we worked on recalling an early feeling of rejection, then discussed it. We concluded that her early sense of rejection has followed her through life, making her feel that she'll never be able to get what she wants because someone else will always get there first. And because she felt that way, we decided, she would unconsciously act in a way to make that situation become true.

"If you understand that and take responsibility for it," I suggested, "perhaps you can turn your life around. You may even hold on to your next job longer."

I invited her to work another week with Dad on the condition that she completes each task perfectly, not for me but for her. After a pause, she agreed.

Hopeful that I had uncovered a truth and that her eyes had been opened to it, I started breakfast while she went to tend to Dad. About ten minutes later, however, she returned full of anger and grabbed her purse.

"I can't do it, Doris. I could do it for you, but not for me!"

"But do it for yourself, Leila Ann, because you gave your word and because you are responsible for the job you do, wherever you are."

She shrugged helplessly and stalked out of the house.

My heart aches, for I see myself in her. Growing up is a long, hard process. Trying to gain the respect of others before you respect yourself is a very difficult task. I'm sad that the pattern is repeating itself again. Another woman fired.

EST 6-DAY

October 1980

I have taken EST Seminars for two years. The two-hour

drive to Miami with other graduates is a mini-seminar in itself during which we share our lives and feelings, and support each other in taking responsibility for creating whatever happens in our lives.

For some time I have watched graduates sharing their experiences of the EST 6-day mountain course and was impressed by the vitality that shone in their faces. Whatever it is, I want it. When I ask them to tell me about the 6-Day Course, they merely smile and say, "Do, it, Doris!"

I have decided to do just that in hopes of getting at the root of my anger and resentment, as I am sure that fear causes anger. And I will have to face my fears if I am to rappel down a mountain, jump off a zip line and pull myself along a rope, belly up across a canyon as in the Tryolean Traverse. I should discover some truths about myself, which could bring a clarity to my life and actions.

Tonight I saw a movie on the 6-Day and was filled with terror. If I had not already decided to take it, I would never have signed up. During the break, I met a charming young woman who looked vaguely familiar. I could not place her until she pulled out photographs of herself taken before and after the 6-Day.

"Don't you remember?" she asked. "We did the Communications Course together." She was transformed. From a shy, awkward teenager, she had matured into a. lovely, secure woman.

I recalled an experience we had shared. Seated in double rows face to face, the "A's" had to choose a partner. "B's" could sit still and be chosen. I had been grateful that I was a "B" and didn't have the responsibility of choosing. When this young woman sat down opposite me, I made a snap judgment that she would be uninteresting. We were told to stare into each other's face for thirty minutes in silence. Suddenly tears rolled down my cheeks. I saw her as a frightened young girl, shy and lonely. I sensed her insecurity, her need to be loved and understood. Her need was my need; I became her.

Afterwards, she told me she had chosen me because I looked so sure of myself. She had always been afraid of those in authority and she wanted to face her fear. It had taken a lot for her to sit down opposite me. We cried together and hugged each other.

Now here she was before me, beautiful and unafraid. Just as she had the initiative to sit opposite me and face what she had feared, she had shown the courage to tackle the 6-Day.

She urged me to do it. "But I'm afraid," I cringed.

"Of course you're afraid," she smiled. "Everyone is. But do it anyway. It was the greatest experience of my life."

When she walked away, I saw that one leg was six inches shorter than the other. My God, I had never even noticed. And still she had the courage to rappel down a mountain. I felt small and insignificant, for now she had become the strong one.

MY PHYSICAL

October 1980

I am almost ready for the six-day. Today I hired Dana and her daughter to take care of Mother and Dad in my absence. They have both worked here separately. They will take turns sleeping on the couch. I feel completely assured that my parents are in good hands.

My physical was fearsome. As I've had high blood pressure in the past, I approached the "stress test" (walking in place until your blood pressure and pulse increase), with great anxiety, fearing my heart might give out.

"I think you had better cancel this EST trip," the cardiologist warned. "You are too anxious and might injure yourself. I can't imagine your having to rappel down a mountain. It's just as wise to make a decision, 'no.' You don't have to do everything. You can make a decision for or against it, and I suggest you don't do it."

My own doctor, however, was supportive. "Go for it, Doris. You need to break away. Do something different. It won't do you any harm. You're not going to die."

And so this dependent child had to make up her own mind and the decision was: "I'll do it!"

ON THE MOUNTAIN

October 1980

There are one hundred people taking the six-day in Kingston, New York. We have classes all day until late at night and often into the early morning. Many of us are living in fear of "The Mountain," as we have not seen it and don't have time to explore.

We fall out at dawn to do exercises on a grassy slope between the cottages. Men and women of all ages, shapes, colors and sizes must participate in the difficult routines. Snow fell on the third day and now we jump and stretch in a large room with mirrors.

Each activity is tightly scheduled and perfectly organized. This is more like the army than the army is. I find myself counting the seconds as I brush my teeth, take a shower and dress. We are constantly reminded of the time by one of the fifty assistants. No one is allowed to wear a watch. We are learning the value of time and what can be accomplished in a minute. I feel I am pitting my life against the elements of time and space.

A WARNING

October 1980

Our leader, hawk-nosed and carping, railed at us today because several people forgot their notebooks.

"You people are going to die on the ropes," he warned. "The class will wait for you to go to your cabin and get your notebooks and pens, but no one will wait for you on The Mountain. It will be life or death. If you can't remember to listen and follow instructions, you will die on the ropes.

"Last year, an older woman had a heart-attack and died in the middle of the Tryolean Traverse (in which you pull yourself across a canyon while dangling from a rope.) Some may think it was our fault, but it was her responsibility."

My terror continues to grow. The tension is thick in the room for we are all guilty of forgetfulness and incompletions. We must face The Mountain because we gave our word. Our lives work, says Werner Erhard, only in so far as we keep our word.

"Do you know that only YOU have responsibility for your lives?" our leader thundered. "And you can't even remember to bring your notebooks! No wonder your world isn't working!"

LETTING GO

October 1980

We are assigned to groups. Mine consists of three women of various ages, two young men, the guide and me. We are huddled in sweaters and jackets against the chill.

We head to the rappel site and I'm pleased, assuming they have given me the easiest task first because they know I'm the oldest, and will have to work up to the difficult one. But then, how do I know which is really the most terrifying? Perhaps it varies with each person.

There was another group before us at the site and we were told to meditate for twenty minutes. I sit cross-legged in a patch of sunlight, gazing at a leaf which turns into a large gaping mouth. The jaws of the mountain are waiting to receive me. A memory comes. I am a child of six pushing my baby brother, Don, in a baby carriage. The carriage overturns as I push it up the curb, and "Donny" falls out. I am afraid I might have killed him. "What did you decide?" I silently ask myself.

"That Mother might think I did it on purpose! That she might never trust me again." Was that why I could not trust others, because I could not trust myself? Even worse, I did not trust others to trust me. Whatever, the word was "trust." I have been living out this lie all my life.

It's time to line up and be fitted for a helmet and harness. A young woman tries to adjust my straps. She seems terribly young. Can I trust her?

"My helmet is too loose, isn't it?" I ask in trepidation. Two girls check me and cannot agree on how it should be adjusted and call in a third. Finally I get another helmet. My God, if they don't know what they're doing, how can I put my trust in them and jump off The Mountain! But I must, even if they are imperfect. God help me!

It's my turn and I step onto a tiny piece of worn green carpet placed on the edge of the cliff. I look down and see jutting rocks and a very steep drop. Fear seizes me. I can envision bits of my flesh stuck to the rocks below. Nobody told me it would be like this. There was no way I could put my body over that edge. Not now—not ever! I felt cheated, trapped. I turned to face my mentor.

"It's scary. I can't do it. No way! Those rocks will kill me!" I blurt wildly.

His eyes blaze. "You gave your word!" I was truly alone with him and The Mountain. I am given two ropes. "The rope in your right hand will act as a brake when you pull it towards your body. The rope in your left hand must slip through your fingers so you can descend. Now, bend your knees and stick out your rear." I did.

"Lean way out over the cliff and take a large step backwards with your right foot, then loosen the rope with your left hand."

`I panicked. This wasn't making any sense. I listened but couldn't hear or understand.

"Wait a minute. Why don't you teach me over there? I promise I'll learn to do it and then I can do it from here." I was bargaining for my life and trying to change the rules. Typical!

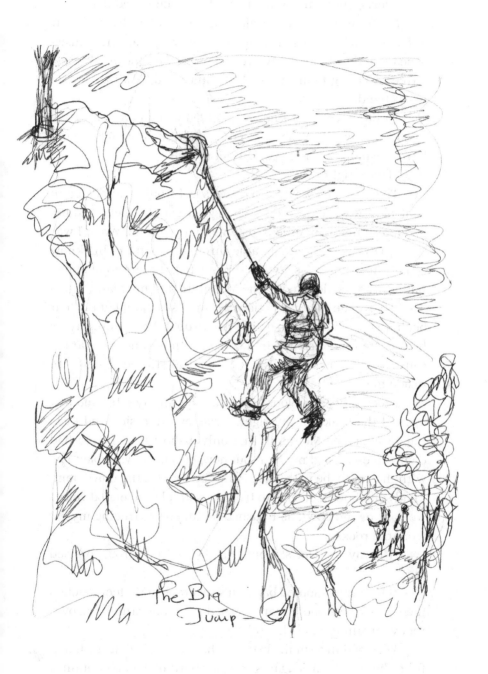

The Big
Jump

"Doris, cut your act and be with me," he yelled fiercely.

My brain froze, jaws rigid, and I could barely talk. Fear as big as three houses enveloped me, leaving me small, insignificant and immobile. My eyes followed the rope as it circled a tree. A young man clutched the other end, holding my life in his hands.

"Wait a minute," I said thickly. "Do you mean that I have to do this myself? You're not going to let me down?" I would have trusted him, perhaps, but not myself.

"That's right."

There was no way out. This was it. I would actually be in control of my own life for a change. It couldn't be! I had depended so much on others to come to my rescue. When I was broke, Daddy and Mother came through. When I didn't know something, there was always somebody out there to help me. But now, I was alone with The Mountain and my fear.

"Give me the instructions again," I said, and felt my fear begin to melt. I meant to do it. I had to do it. Now, strangely, as he repeated the instruction, I could listen beyond my fear because my fear became so small that it was stuffed somewhere inside me.

I took a big step, loosening the rope in my left hand as I opened the brake in my right. I was over the side and kicking away at The Mountain that only a short time before had owned me—owned my fear. But now, because I was able to be with the youth, be with The Mountain, be with the movement, I had somehow been able to trust myself. I heard elated voices welcoming me down as I pushed out in space, freeing myself from the rocks.

"Hooray for Doris! Come on, Doris!" my group praised me.

"I love it!" I shouted back. "It's so simple!" My feet touched the rocks below and I nearly turned my ankle stumbling over rocky terrain to reach the others.

We stood in a small clearing, sharing my joy—just a handful of human beings against the strength of The Mountain. I felt huge and capable of flying. We turned to support our seventh member.

All agreed that this was the most frightening experience we had ever encountered in our entire life. We then proceeded single file through the woods towards our second site.

THE ZIP LINE

I climb a tall ladder up to a flat wooden platform built completely around a tree. I must jump from this gallows, but I can't imagine having the courage. Strange, I think. It's like birth; the women prepare us and the men catch us. Or like dying and being born again. It's all a game, but why would anyone want to play it? What does it prove? My fears threaten to overwhelm me as I reach the top step. Two steady hands clasp my shoulders and I look into a pair of calm blue eyes and the clear oval face of a young blonde woman.

"Doris, are you afraid?"

"Yes," I gasp. "I guess so!"

"Just listen to the instructions and do what he tells you. It's as simple as that."

"OK. I'll try." I nod bravely and edge around the tree growing through the platform. There is no railing and I have ten inches to shimmy by, twenty feet off the ground. A stalwart youth in a red jacket, with sea-green eyes, greets me. He orders me to look down. My eyes take in the lake far below, the distant trees and the small group of men waiting for me at the water's edge.

"It's very high!" Again my fear envelops me. Must I step off this safe platform and zoom down on a rope towards the waiting men?

"See that iron bar above your head? You are going to grab it and step off the platform." He fastens me into a safety-harness. I am alone again. Why am I here, demanding of myself that I conquer this fear, own it? Will it be owned for all time?

Will I allow fear to overpower me in the future if I conquer this now? I must meet my own fear—or meet my death.

"Look down again. What do you see? How do you feel?" He is asking me to observe myself as I am observing. So this is how it's done! Watch yourself as you go through the trauma. How do you react? What do you feel? Will this make it easier—setting yourself apart from it? If I step away from my problems in caring for Mom and Dad, will I be better able to handle them?

I look down again. Gentle, green trees and a cerulean lake! It's beautiful, I suddenly realize. Why should I be afraid? I belong to it and it belongs to me. I am a part of it all.

"Nature is beautiful," I whisper in awe.

"Step to the edge of the platform." His voice holds me like a vise. "Grab the iron bar and don't let go until you are told to." He clips me into place. "Keep your back straight. One ... two ... three, go!"

I grab the bar. I don't look into the abyss but keep my eyes on the goal. My heart is hammering. I'll do it! I'll do it! I'll publish my book on India, "It's Not Too Far." It's not too far for me to go from here to there. I'll do it alone!

But I don't step boldly into space. Instead, my knees fold under me and I quietly glide away until suddenly I am like a giant bird dangling from the wire, dancing in space. I sing and shout, "I love it! I love it!"

The thrill of the zip line is all too short. My feet touch earth and I forget the instructions, immediately letting go of the bar. Four men pounce on me to unclip the rope, and I stagger across the rough ground to join my group.

TYROLEAN TRAVERSE

From the trail we can see two forms hanging upside down from a rope extending across a canyon. We stand still for several minutes, appalled at the fact that the furthest figure is immobile. We are sent to the woods to meditate. As I sit, I wonder if I, too, will be stuck. As I stare at the leaves, an eye comes into view. Who is it, I wonder? And why do I see only part of a face?

Again we line up for our gear. I am fitted with a helmet and harness and told to walk to the ridge and stand alone under an isolated, gray tree. The tree makes me think of Christ. He was nailed to a cross of wood. I am to pull myself across this canyon, hand over hand, until I reach the other side.

Two assistants prepare to send one of our group across. He is suspended from the rope by a cable attached to his harness like an umbilical cord, his legs sprawling to the side like a baby in a crib. I remember a baby monkey I saw outside the Taj Mahal clinging upside down to its mother's belly. There is something fetal about this position, reminding one that birth and death are part of the same coin.

The youth starts across and I look over the raw edge of the cliff into the canyon, its floor all sharp rocks and muddy flowing water. No one facing the crossing can see the canyon until they reach this tree. There is time to look down and backwards at one's life. As the youth moves towards the center, pulling himself slowly hand over hand, people on the other side shout encouragement.

Tears well within me. Surely my arms won't be strong enough to pull my body the last twenty feet. Would I live to get to the other side? Somewhere deep in my soul, I am sure that this is the end of my life. I have brought my parents just so far and now I am giving up. It is impossible to support them any longer, for I cannot face their eventual deaths. Therefore I won't make it. I don't have the strength, or perhaps, the will.

My God! I suddenly realize that there are forty people here helping me get to the other side of The Mountain. My parents only have me to help them get to the other side of life and I lack the will to do it. What kind of a person am I that I can't even help them face their own demise ... that I must run from reality like I run from my own death? I feel so small and unworthy. Would they ever forgive me? Tears flow down my cheeks as huge sobs rack my body. "Oh, my God. Oh, Jesus, please forgive me for I am not worthy."

"Doris!" My name rings out and I stumble blindly towards the ropes. "Pull down the wire," a young woman orders, ignoring my tears. After some fumbling I find it and pull it down. She attaches it to me. Again fear claims me, but when I push off, I am no longer afraid. This time it is easy. I will be all right!

In the center of the rope, I let go and spread my arms out like an eagle, sprawling in space high above the rocky abyss many feet below. I look down and think, "This is perfect trust. I trust the ropes, the assistants, myself."

In the last twenty feet when the going gets tough, I begin to use both hands to pull my body upward. I dread the difficult part, when I must pit my strength, my breath, my life, against the ropes—against gravity. I think of the things that are incomplete in my life. "I can do it," I yell.

"Hooray for Doris," my group chants. "You can do it!" Those who have successfully crossed are clapping me on.

Clasping the rope with both hands and heaving my body upwards inch by inch, I shout to the universe: "I can do it! I can do it!" I can sell my songs, perform a one-woman show, publish a book, exhibit my paintings!

Then I have arrived amidst a great hubbub. When I have been unbuckled, I fall into a stranger's arms. "Oh, my God!" I wail in despair, tears streaming down my cheeks. "I never thought of my parents once!"

Strong arms embrace me, holding me tight. The stranger is suddenly a father figure, his arms symbolizing all of the love and support I have just received from people on both sides of the canyon.

"Perhaps you've learned something," the stranger says. At this moment he is no longer a stranger. He is me.

"Yes. I have to think of me before I think of them. Or I can't really love them or feel loved by them. I have to be me."

I melt into the crowd of EST graduates, all people who are

willing to give their word and keep it, people who believed in the best in me. How grateful I am to these assistants who are helping us to be born again, born into new knowledge of what is really true for us.

Is this the answer I have been searching for? "I must do unto others as I would have them do unto me." And in order to know what to do for them, I have to first be kind to myself, consider myself worthy, able, knowledgeable, beautiful, loved.

In order to be loving you must first feel loved. Certainly! But who is to blame for my not feeling loved, feeling shut out? Are we not responsible for everything that happens to us? I saw the eye again, and the anguished mouth, the deep cry of a child wanting its mother, wanting to know it wasn't alone in the night ... wanting protection, security, love.

Were not my parents also like little children? I could hear the great wail that rose from the depths of my paralyzed father, alone and afraid. And Mother, who like the little bird trying to help its injured mate, was helpless to carry the burden alone.

I, too, have been unable to make it alone, unable to cross this abyss, unable to carry the great burden of two parents becoming my children. Was I really alone? And could I carry this responsibility? I had been resisting and what you resist persists. I knew now that the blame and resentment I held against my parents for not showing love and respect all came from me. I was their child. Of course they loved me. But somehow I had interpreted it all wrong.

Now I knew I could do it, could be myself. I knew also that I was not alone, for they, in their aloneness, were also me. We could do it together. It takes a team to support each individual. I had to be part of a team. I had to open my eyes, my heart, my life, to what lay ahead, and not be afraid.

I had faced a steep cliff and found a safe way to rappel to earth. I had taken the zip line, making a quick diagonal descension, taking my whole self with me, hurling my body upon the loving trust and acceptance of others. And I had crossed the canyon, experiencing the horizontal rope from man to man, crossing the bridge of acceptance, crossing from the unknown to the known, crossing from the anguish of pain and terror and daily burdens to the other side of the mountain.

"What are you going to leave on The Mountain?" our guide asked us as we shared our experiences of the Tryolean Traverse.

"I don't want to leave anything behind," I blurted passionately. Typical. Whenever I travel, I gather moss and take it with me—costumes, paintings, music, writing. "I want to carry The Mountain with me, take it in my pocket. It is something I never want to forget. Something to cherish ... always."

The Mountain is within us, I thought. It is not out there to be crossed, leaped from, or mounted, but it is our awakening, our summit. It is to have it all inside you and to be the clearing, the space between mountains, to be the jump, the fall, the height. To have all passion, all fear, all hope, all love within you and to know that all mankind has the same within.

We are all stumbling, fumbling, fearful and angry in our search for perfection, harmony, love and peace. If only we open our eyes, the distance from me to you is as short as the blink of an eye. It is understanding, insight and compassion. It is perhaps, knowing, as Werner Erhard says, that it is a "you *and* me" world. And that it doesn't work when we behave as if it is a "you *or* me" world.

Tomorrow we will share aloud with our group of one hundred. And, amazingly, it has been reported that all one hundred of us have succeeded in keeping our word. We have conquered The Mountain.

October 1980

Arriving home after the 6-Day, I rushed into my mother's bedroom and tried to tell her about my experience on The

Mountain. It was 9 p.m. and she was nearly asleep. I shared my fears and my discoveries, telling her that I now realized it wasn't her fault that I had thought she and Dad didn't love me, but that I was responsible for this mistaken belief. I guess I thought I was absolving her from her sins.

She did not comprehend. I had conquered The Mountain, but I had again failed in life. What was going wrong? I let all of the fear overtake me again, fear of The Mountain. This was still my mountain, communicating with my mother.

I fled to the living room, unable to breathe and more exhausted than I had ever been in my life. All of the pressures of time and space caught up with me. I recalled the time we had jogged up a hill. A couple of hundred feet into the run, two assistants greeted me, goading me on.

"Run, Doris, run. Don't stop now. You can make it. You've only just begun. Go!" I stood there completely out of breath and bawling like a baby. Me, over fifty, facing these youngsters ordering me up The Mountain over a trail studded with rocks. It wasn't enough that I had come this far. I had to keep going. Every two hundred feet or so, I found the assistants, cold, heartless and inhuman, goading me on. How I had wished I could take these little EST gremlins home with me to sit on my desk when I was stuck with my writing.

"Don't stop! Don't look back! Don't get into your head! Don't let one thought deter you from your goal! Don't look down! Look only where you are going! Look at the goal!" I know now why Lot's wife was turned into a pillar of salt when she looked back at the burning city.

Now my body was rebelling. Surely I would die. Not on The Mountain, but here in the safety and comfort of my parent's home. Now who was writing the script? Had I caused this? But I didn't want to die. No way! I called the hospital and spoke to a nurse in Emergency.

"The blood is rushing up my body and I'm going to die. I'm afraid! What shall I do?"

"Put your head between your knees. Now, is there anyone else in the house?" she asked.

"My mother," I gasped. "She's in the other room. Oh, please, let me hang up and you call her back to come in here and help me!" I couldn't go to her and I was afraid to be alone. I needed support. I was at the bottom of the canyon and I had to get to the other side.

Mother came in after the nurse's phone call, and I lay in a ball on the floor. She got me some tea. I kept my head down and tried to breathe calmly. Finally we both went to bed. I had fought the demon of fear one more time. But I had still not communicated.

DISCOVERY

December 1980

Since the 6-Day, I have become involved in the Hunger Project aimed at ending hunger in the world. It has taught me that what looms as a large personal problem becomes small when you take on a greater task. Somehow the problem of Dad's stroke takes its place on the back burner and my life assumes a new perspective. All of my talents in writing, dance and theater can be directed towards helping create harmony, peace and fulfillment in the world.

I somehow have less patience for Dad now, even though I had expected to have more. I want him to cross the canyon, too. I wonder if I am different. I think probably I am more *me* than I ever was before. I have become larger and my parents smaller in my own eyes. I no longer lie down and let them walk on me. Perhaps I can take them with me. Ah, that's it. We are a team. We are in it together.

And hope above hope, I have heard there is a Stroke Club in Stuart. Perhaps I can help to nurture, develop and contribute to it. That which is wanted and needed has come about, and will harbor new stroke couples so that they may profit from each other's experience.

INSIDE JOB

January 1981

Our newest aide showed up at 8 a.m. today. She is a short, plump, black woman I found through a service agency. She has worked in a nursing home and has had experience with stroke patients, the agency told me. And, they said, she desperately needs a job.

We were matched on that point because I desperately needed an aide. I had been on duty alone for several weeks and had not received any answers to my advertisements for a new aide.

The new aide appeared cooperative and knowledgeable. She watched me exercise Dad, and when I started his shower, she offered to take over. She then dressed and walked him, and I was enormously pleased. I felt she was an answer to my prayers and I could already envision her working here for six months or more.

I had an appointment at noon and she offered to stay on to fix lunch and leave at 1 p.m., locking up after herself. I left my parents and house in her care and went to my appointment.

When I returned at 4 p.m., I opened the silver drawer to prepare for cocktails and was stunned to find Mom's sterling silver gone. My first thought, of course, was that "Suzy" had taken it. I called the sheriff's department and they promised to send a deputy around the next day.

Mother was crestfallen. "I've had that silver since the day I was married," she said tearfully. "It was given to me by my mother." I can understand her sense of loss, but I don't put so much feeling into the possession of things that can tarnish, wear out, or get stolen. They are beautiful while we have them. And we identify with them so that when we lose them, we feel that a part of ourselves is gone. I have little use for silver, antiques, furs or jewelry. To me, it is far more important to have long grass, high shrubs, untamed trees and wild birds in my yard.

January 1981

I was nervous about going to bed last night for fear that the thief might return and I double locked the doors. At 3 a.m., Dad let out a blood-curdling scream and I leaped from my bed. I found him in his room, wild eyed and pointing frantically towards the kitchen.

The kitchen door leading to the garage was unlocked. Could I possibly have left it open? The kitchen radio was gone and I found a pile of our possessions on the garage floor: a Talking Book record player (not really much use to a thief as it won't play ordinary records), a tape recorder, and a heater. The garage door was partly open and the screen in the window above Dad's workbench had been pushed in.

"Good for you, Dad," I said when I returned to the bedroom. "You have good ears." I assumed that he had heard a noise or seen a light in the garage. I felt that his screams had probably driven away the thieves before they could escape with the loot.

Dad was raving with rage and fear at this assault on his home and possessions. His terror was undoubtedly multiplied by his own sense of helplessness. I gave him some milk and a tranquilizer.

I wondered if Suzy had returned with friends to rob us. Next morning the sheriff's deputy was puzzled by the pushed-in screen over the workbench. The window was the jalousie type and the thieves couldn't have entered through it.

I was very disturbed by the incident and my sense of trust has been severely weakened.

* * *

Suzy came back to work and appeared surprised to hear about the robbery. She immediately disclaimed any responsibility.

"If I had done it, why would I have come to work today?" she asked.

I told her that I thought it had to be more than a coincidence that the silver disappeared the first day she had been here. She grew quite upset at my accusations and threatened to leave. I told her to stay or I would be positive that she had taken the silver. I wanted her here when the sheriff's deputy returned. She stayed, grumbling.

When the deputy arrived, she became distraught. "I didn't take that silver! I ain't no thief!"

I asked the deputy to search her house, and Suzy became enraged. "You can't come to my house. I got children and I won't have you messing up my things. I won't let you go to my house, when I didn't do no stealing." She turned and gave me a truculent look: "You think you got trouble, girl? I'll show you trouble."

The deputy spoke with her awhile and then told me that there was nothing he could do. Helpless and angry, I paid Suzy off, convinced that she was guilty and getting away with it

THE GIRDLE

January 1981

We drove Don to the airport today. He will be flying to Taiwan shortly to study Chinese art. What an exciting life he has and how I would love to be free again to travel, as in my show-business days. I am frankly jealous of his freedom; while I sit here watching two parents disintegrate as they rub against each other like polished stones. Although the experience can be fruitful, it is also painful.

Dad smiled through tears as Don kissed him goodbye. I briefly clasped my brother's taut, bird-strength to my bosom. He is gone.

I leave my parents to console each other. I can't bear to watch Dad's sadness turn into frustration and finally belligerence. He and Don have gained a closeness that is beautiful to see. I have often envied my brother's ability to make Dad laugh and communicate. It's so foreign to Dad's nature to act the compliant, affable person that he is with Don. I know that he loves his son very much.

I return to walk Dad to the car. Again he has become my child, the umbilical cord of his illness tying him to me. We must learn from our parents how to walk into the darkness. In their suffering, they teach us how to march towards death. I never cease to wonder about the perfect design of life as created by our Maker. Although we "kick against the pricks" (Acts, 9, vs. 5) and try to "spit the bit out of our mouth" (James, 3, vs. 3), this is the direction we must take to our next destination.

As we near Palm Beach on the way back from the airport, Mother mentions that she would like to stop and buy a girdle.

"We'll turn off here and go to the mall," I suggest. I have long looked askance at her ancient tattered girdle that she pulls on every morning. She cannot go without her stockings.

Dad begins raving and shaking his head no. "Now, Dad, don't be selfish," I reprimand. "Mother needs a girdle and you can sit in the car, walk around the mall, or go to the men's room if you wish."

I start to turn off the road and am horrified when Dad grabs the wheel, veering the Chrysler back into the traffic lane. My heart sinks with fear as we narrowly miss a car behind us. This is the last straw! I have tried to be gentle with two people who are absorbing my life, but I do not want to lose my life because of Dad's whims.

"Dad, you nearly killed us," I hiss venomously. "If you ever touch this wheel again, I shall never take you out in this car as long as I live!"

I have pulled to the side of the road. The sky is a huddled mass of clouds, which let forth a torrential downpour. Livid with anger, I back up to the intersection through the blinding rain.

Fast! If he could take chances with my life, I could take chances with his.

I reach in the back seat for my orange poncho, yank it over my head and jump out, slamming the door behind me in a fever of hate, abandoning my parents at the intersection. I stalk away into the rain, farther and farther, until I can no longer see them. I want to walk out of their lives—forever.

I have left them to think. I am sick of playing victim. Sick of being used. Sick of doing all of the work and being considered the "bad" one, no matter what I do. I stay away, hoping that they are suffering. Hoping that they are afraid.

Somewhere in the deluge I make the decision: I want to be treated like a person; I want my own room. Am I important to them? If I am, then I shall treat myself as if I were. I shall begin to respect myself and maybe they will respect me. I shall start to make decisions. Dad has always held a strange power over me, casting fear over my soul. And Mother calls the shots. She is a "No" person. Well, it's time I took the reins.

I walk back slowly, very slowly, tasting the sweetness of revenge. I am fighting for my life. Fighting the very people who have given me birth. Strange how the tables turn. The mountains become leveled and the valleys filled.

I open the door. Mother is trying to console Dad.

"Doris, where did you go? Why did you do that? You left us sitting here in the middle of traffic! It's dangerous. You're upsetting Dad." Terror lay beneath her words. I have punished her but she has done nothing to me. Too furious to speak, I drive home in silence, my anger draining me of every particle of energy. Exhausted, I fling myself on the couch and let Mother put Dad to bed.

Just before dozing off, I vaguely hear the words, "Doris, if you ever pull a stunt like that again, I will never allow you to drive our car as long as I live." Her anger echoes mine. A slow smile spreads over my face as I recognize the same words with which I had threatened Dad. Our anguish is a three-way power struggle. All of this hate, anger, revenge and silent treatment is so childish. Will we never grow up? We nearly lost our lives today over a silly girdle.

I fell asleep knowing that we three prisoners are damned lucky to be alive.

* * *

The next day I told Dad that I felt I needed a bed and asked if he would like to go back in with Mother and let me move into the guest room. He would be giving up a lot—a private bath, a view of the birds that come to the feeder, a private room. He shook his head emphatically "no." I wondered how I could steal a room out from under his body.

I called our minister in desperation. When he came to visit, he observed how Mother and I were at loggerheads. "You've met your equal, Doris. Your mother will never give up. All you can do is to give in gracefully."

"I'll never give up."

"Then one or both of you will continue to be miserable."

Later, over "cocktails," he asked Dad casually, "Bob, would you be willing to move into your own room with Polly so Doris can have a room by herself? She's doing a lot to help out, you know, and she doesn't have a room."

Dad shook his head from side to side.

"Well," the minister continued. "Would you be willing to move if you could have your hospital bed?"

Dad nodded yes.

I was flabbergasted. How clever! I had never thought of the fact that Dad would want his own bed. Poor Dad! How difficult for him to communicate what he feels to two dumb females, who can't even ask the right question.

I could barely contain my elation. At last, after nearly five years, I would be considered one of the family again. No more sleeping on the hard couch or in a hot garage. I could have my own room and I could work in my leisure time on my writing. No more carrying a typewriter back and forth or being at the mercy of the weather.

Oh, bless you, Mr. P.

January, 1981

Peter, a friend who works as a hospital aide, called today and I asked him to help me move Dad's bed into Mother's bedroom. He agreed, and promised to bring a friend.

They were here within the hour and I told Dad what they were going to do. I expected him to renege or put up a fuss, but he was completely passive.

It was not an easy job, requiring a lot of dismantling, but eventually it was done. The hospital bed was in Mom and Dad's room and the twin bed was now in what was to be my room. This was the room I had used as a visitor thirty years ago before Dad bought me the house in Stuart. What a lot has happened since then.

I feel somehow that I am the crippled one, and I won't become whole until I am alone in the world. When will that be? Will there be any time left for me? This, at least, is a start and I can begin to feel all of a piece.

I am thrilled to have a room of my own and have begun to move Dad's clothes into Mom's closet and my things in from the garage. I shall put my bed against the North wall so I can lie in the North-South direction which yogis believe contributes to a more healthy sleep. Why didn't I do this years ago? It will take some adjustment. Dad will be farther away from the bathroom and he will probably still have to use my bathroom, as it has a shower and there is a grab bar by the commode.

Mom's room is very beautiful, all in blues, with a lovely baby-blue rug and bedspreads, blue walls, flowered drapes, a long wooden headboard that Dad constructed, and beige furniture. From his bed, Dad will now be able to look out on the river.

MOM'S COAT

February 3, 1981

My rage at mother is grounded in fear, as her mind is slipping. I lost my temper today when I discovered that her aqua coat was filthy. It has become my responsibility to see that her clothes are clean. But isn't it enough to take care of Dad?

I had put Dad in the car and returned to the house for my pocketbook and list, when I heard Dad cry out. I found Mother lying on the concrete by the garage door, which had been left half open. I was afraid she'd had a stroke. Yet she was calling my name.

"Quick, Doris, help me get up."

"What happened, Mother?"

"Oh, my arm! Please move me. My arm hurts." I decided not to move her and called an ambulance. I returned to calm Dad.

"Oh, Doris, I'm so cold, so cold!" Mother cried. I grabbed a piece of rug and slid it carefully under her frail body and then wrapped her in a blanket.

The ambulance attendants gave her oxygen and slid her gently onto a stretcher. "She's probably broken her arm. We'll put it in an air sling and take her to the hospital," the paramedic said.

I prepared a quick sandwich for Dad and we followed closely behind. I left Dad in the coffee shop with his sandwich, and hurried to Emergency.

"Oh, Doris, thank God you've come. I'm freezing." I covered her with a blanket and told her Dad and I would pick her up as soon as the doctor had seen her.

"I'm sorry this happened, Mom. It was stupid of me to leave the garage door half open." Apparently she had tried unsuccessfully to duck under it. It was also stupid of me to have lost my temper, I might have added. Guilt hung over me like a dark cloud.

DOUBLE DUTY

February 4, 1981

Mom's arm was broken and now I have two patients instead of one. They put her arm in a sling, rather than a cast, so it is difficult for her to move without hurting it. Dad agreed to let her use his hospital bed so she can punch a button and rise up to a sitting position. I must help her get out of bed, wash, and dress.

At night I make a bed of pillows and sleep on the floor in the hall outside their room. I waken several times a night to help her go to the bathroom (she has only one kidney).

Dad is upset about losing his hospital bed but he is very concerned about Mom and is actually considerate for a change. When I am dressing her, he helps me do up her sweater. He asks her to walk with him and she tags behind with her right finger in his belt. I don't know who is walking whom.

The other day Mom helped Dad do up his pants and nearly fell. He is much taller than she is and I fear a double fall. If they go down together something else may break.

DAD'S PANTS

February 10, 1981

I have been angry and frustrated at Dad for not learning to dress himself. He refuses to cooperate in helping me do up his pants, for example, when he makes his many trips to the bathroom. And I have been afraid to have Mom help him, as they might fall together again. After all, she is more fragile since she broke her arm.

Today I made desperate and futile calls to Home Health. There are no occupational therapists available, who could help him learn to dress himself. Such training would not fall under Medicare for some strange reason. I feel it is just as important to learn activities of daily living as it is to have a physical therapist teach him how to exercise.

We do have a pamphlet put out by the American Heart Association on how to teach a stroke patient to dress himself in bed, but I haven't been successful in getting Dad to cooperate. Possibly it is more difficult for a member of the family to teach these things. I am stymied because Mother still won't let me take him to the Rehabilitation Center in Palm Beach.

Perhaps I could get him a pair of the Indian-style pants we use in yoga classes that come with a draw string rather than a zipper. He might be able to pull them up by himself. At least, it would be easier for Mother to help him.

February 12, 1981

Ah, victory! The drawstring pants idea led me to a sports store this afternoon and I picked up a very beautiful jogging suit of rust velour with straight legs and a diagonal black stripe across the front of the jacket.

It fits Dad perfectly and I'm thrilled. A tan wool cap tops off the outfit and he looks positively stunning. The paralyzed arm fits snugly underneath the zippered jacket. Dad made the rounds in his new outfit and he looks so handsome I am proud of him.

This will help in the bathroom as he can lean against the wall and pull up the left side of his pants while a helper pulls up the right.

February 16, 1981

For some reason Dad will no longer wear the jogging suit and I'm angry and frustrated. It had worked well and he had seemed pleased. Mom has been able to help him and I can go to EST. I'm now involved in the Hunger Project aimed at ending world hunger by the year 2000. Either we intend to use bombs to blow ourselves up, or we will start to care about each other, and spend our efforts alleviating lack, sharing food, and spending money where it can save lives instead of destroying them. If we can get enough committed people in the world, it can be done. Thousands of people have signed a pledge to contribute time, talent, money and prayers to ending hunger—as an "idea whose time has come."

Today I did something I shall never forgive myself for. Dad and I were in the bathroom and I was trying to help him pull his pants up. He wouldn't cooperate and I lost my temper.

"Dad, I do not want to have to pull up your pants for the next twenty years!" His face registered shock and disbelief, and I could have bitten out my tongue. Had I given up on him? Didn't I care any more?

"I mean, Dad. I think you can help me. I'm involved with the Hunger Project and I need time and cooperation to be able to work on it. There are millions of people who are starving . . ."

It was too much for him to comprehend. All he really understood was that I had withdrawn my support. I am heartsick.

APHASIC FRIEND

February 18, 1981

For several years now I have envisioned starting a Stroke Club. Last week I heard that seven stroke couples have been meeting at the Martin County Library once a month for a year. Thrilled, I called the president and founder, whose husband is also aphasic and cannot talk.

Today we were invited to visit them at their trailer. Tom, a ruddy, smiling man with sandy hair and a slight limp, met us at the door. He ushered Dad to a flowered love seat and proceeded to use sign language, asking Dad how long ago since he had his stroke. We women helped the men communicate. Tom pulled out a red photo album and asked Dad if he would like to see it.

"Photography is Tom's hobby," explained his wife. "He's really very good although he does it only for fun." Photographs of a child's face, a flower, an old fisherman and some water scenes were much appreciated by Dad, whose eyes lit up like a schoolboy's.

"Dad taught me how to enlarge and develop prints," I interjected eagerly. As an artist I appreciated the excellent quality of Tom's compositions and color. He took several pictures of Dad. How I wish Dad had some activity or talent which would occupy him and of which he could be proud. I am just happy, however, that he is doing well and can walk alone, holding his head up, and is interested in his surroundings.

We were served tea and cake and the "strokers" seemed to appreciate each other without talking. How many men, I thought, are not very emotional until they get a stroke, and then their personal emotions are revealed in a way that was never evident before. Dad's experience of another aphasic, I am sure, makes him feel less alone in the world. What a pity that five years have passed before he had the opportunity to meet another patient with the same disease.

Dad sat on the couch and appeared interested and alive, with a trace of his old humility and graciousness, grateful to be invited to their home. Tom was an inspiration. He urged Dad to climb the two steps into their living room, discarding his cane. He had never done this before. We have not taken him to the Indian River Drive Club luncheons because we did not think he could mount the steps. Mother has gone alone. But today Dad surprised me by handing me his cane and grabbing the rail with his good arm. He pulled himself up step by step, and I returned his cane at the top step.

I am overjoyed that we have at last found a stroke club we can attend, and I will do what I can to publicize the next meeting. I'm sure there are others in Martin County, who are just as alone and suffering the devastating results of stroke. They must be reached as soon as possible.

Upon leaving, a neighbor came over for a jump and I walked to Tom's van to help him remove the jumper cable.

"Here, let me help you," I offered. He gave me a quick punch in the belly, much to my astonishment, which hurt! My shock turned to anger until I evaluated the situation. Here was another "stroker," like Dad, whose anger could also be easily aroused when you tried to help him. "This goes with the disease," I told myself. Out loud I apologized for trying to help.

But the punch in the stomach was well worth the visit.

PART SIX

FINAL VICTORY

(February 1981 - March 1981)

VI

STROKE CLUB MEETING

February 19, 1981

Today Mom, Dad and I attended our first Stroke Club meeting at the library in Stuart. I had sent publicity releases to several newspapers and was thrilled to see forty stroke victims and their spouses parading in, the strokers with canes, on crutches, or in wheelchairs.

The three of us sat in the back. When a neurologist began to speak on the cause and effect of stroke, Dad bawled so loudly that Mother and I had to escort him out of the room.

After the meeting, I invited several stroke-aphasic victims and their spouses to meet Dad. They are lovely people. One aphasic has a big grin and seems anxious to communicate. I look forward to having them visit in the near future. Stephen, an attractive elderly gentleman, approached me.

"I lost my wife to cancer three months ago," he said, eyes brimming with tears. I clasped his hand firmly, feeling his deep loneliness.

"We need you," I said. "My father is an aphasic and can't talk, but he enjoys visitors. Would you be willing to come and visit us in Jensen?"

"I'd love to," he said eagerly. "I came here because I had to talk to someone," he confided, crying again. "I have some beautiful slides of flowers and sunsets. Can I bring them to show your father?"

I consented and his eyes lit up. He will come next Friday.

A WARNING

February 25, 1981

Mother commented that Dad hasn't been too aware for the past few days, although I hadn't noticed anything unusual.

"He's unable to concentrate," she said. "He doesn't seem to be able to understand when I'm reading to him and I'm worried."

It's true. Sometimes he doesn't respond at all to our questions and even the customary "Wa-wa-wa's" have disappeared. When I asked him if he wanted to go to Jensen with me, he shook his head, "No." That was unusual because he usually welcomes a chance to drive downtown. I felt the old tinge of rejection, and wondered whether he was angry at me, or just wasn't feeling well.

I shouted goodbye to Mom and went out. After a few steps, I stopped, startled to hear an inner voice saying clearly: "Doris, you had better say goodbye to your father now, because soon you won't be able to." Where had the voice come from? Why this frightening admonition? Surely there was no possibility that he was near death—or was he?

I felt guilty that I hadn't said goodbye and realized as I walked through the porch, that I would miss him when he was gone. Yes, I would actually miss helping him into the car, lifting the heavy foot, and driving in quiet togetherness along Indian River Drive, a lovely two-lane road bordering the river and one of the most beautiful drives in Florida.

I thought about his sharp "Huh-huh-huh's" when I drove too fast. He would point angrily to the speedometer.

"I'll go slow when we approach the village, Dad," I promised him, but he would continue roaring until I slowed down.

Perhaps his weak eye made if difficult for him to see the whole road from a moving car.

Turning abruptly, I walked back into the living room. Dad was seated in the old, brown chair, his head slumped on his chest. Was he ill? If only he could tell us what was wrong, but the dull, glazed look seemed to come from another place.

"Goodbye, Dad," I said. He raised his head slowly, acknowledging me with a brief nod. "Are you sure you don't want to go downtown with me?" I asked again. A distant, abstract look crossed his face. Again he shook his head, no.

February 27, 1981

Stephen, the man from the stroke club, came at 7 p.m. and set up his screen. Although somewhat dazed and uncomfortable, Dad gave the slides his full attention, gasping in admiration at the glowing colors of nature—a red rose glistening with dew drops, yellow forsythias against a white house, flaming autumn leaves against a cerulean sky.

The pictures reflected a lifetime of memories for Stephen and there were several photos of his late wife. I wondered what treasured incidents Dad and Mother recalled from their travels to Greece, Italy, Switzerland, Norway, Sweden and England. The vibrant colors exuded a healing quality, charging the room with emotion and the awareness of time present, past and future. The slides captured the fragile quality of life and depicted the transient order and perfection of nature in its seasonal splendor, progressing from birth to death to birth.

At eight, Dad's bedtime, he scrunched forward in his chair and reached for his cane. He made his adieus to Stephen, stretching out his arm in thanks. I helped him to rise and walked him into the bedroom. Mother thanked Stephen and retired to dress Dad for bed.

Thrilled at the beauty of these glowing slides and glad that they had awakened in Dad a partial response, I suggested to Stephen that he take his presentation to residents in nursing homes, which might be valuable therapy for him, as well.

Thank you, Lord, for our second friend whom we met through the stroke club.

During the night, I was awakened three times by loud howling. Dad was enveloped in pain, tears of agony rolling down his cheeks.

"Dad, tell me where it hurts," I pleaded. No answer. He could not understand the words or connect the words to the pain. I placed my hand on different parts of his abdomen, but the gesture was futile. He could not grasp the meaning of the word "where." He did understand the word hospital and shook his head no each time.

The next day I canceled a trip to Miami and took a brief morning swim at Jensen Beach. I called Mother every half-hour to see how Dad was. He had no more pain during the day and the evening, too, was quiet.

March 1, 1981

The pain returned with a vengeance this morning. Dad woke crying uncontrollably and we took him to the hospital. We sat three hours in the waiting room while Dad groaned in agony. Finally tests were taken and the doctors could find nothing. He was given a catheter and we were told to go home and give him some pills for the bladder.

March 3, 1981

Dad has not been eating and he can barely walk, even with assistance. I went to an EST Seminar in Miami with a friend. The warning from my internal voice had frightened me and I wanted to establish communication with Dad before it was too late.

I confided my troubles to a young man named Ralph. Shy and withdrawn before he took the EST Training, Ralph had dissolved barriers of fear, mistrust and resentment and blossomed into a physically appealing, and mentally buoyant individual.

"Ralph," I asked in anguish. "Why can't I break through to

my father? Why do I still feel he rejects me? I want to know why I feel my father doesn't love me. I can't ask him because it wouldn't be fair. He could only say "Wa-wa."

"Is Dad's anger real?" I went on. "Does he hate me and do I hate him? Why can't I tell him I love him? And do I love him?"

"Doris, you've got to go back in time to when you first felt his rejection," Ralph counseled, "for you are the one who created that, and you are the only one who can uncreate it."

"It goes back to birth, then," I said. "From the beginning, I felt as if he did not want me around, as though I were interrupting something. He was so happy with Mother that he wasn't ready for a baby. He wanted her all to himself. He and his mother were unable to show affection and he married a woman who radiates warmth and love."

"Aha!" I said with sudden insight. "Dad has been like her child since he's been sick. Perhaps that's the problem. All of his life he watched us children receiving her affection and now it's his turn and he wants it all. Again, I am in the way."

"And you created that!" Ralph said mercilessly.

I remembered the time at the cottage in Maine, when I had been angry at my parents because there was no place downstairs for my belongings. I had felt then that there was no place for me. Now there was no time for me. I felt as if nothing had changed in my life—only my anxiety, which had increased due to Dad's illness.

* * *

Dad woke at 7:30 a.m. the next morning, anxious to go to the bathroom. I hastily dressed him in socks, shoes and his maroon robe and walked him to the bathroom. When he reached the hallway, his paralyzed leg contracted in a spasm and the tall body leaned against me like a sinking ship. With Mother's help I managed to get him seated on the toilet where he collapsed against the wall.

I offered him two laxative pills, which he swept violently aside. I helped him to stand. He was extremely tipsy and Mother helped me walk him into the Florida room. Folding the lanky body into his elevated chair, I observed the sweating forehead. Mother stood behind him supporting his head and crooning words of comfort. I watched dumbfounded as the color drained slowly from his face. I felt as if I had lived this moment before.

"People are just like leaves," a voice in my head said. "They change color before they fall!"

I hastily called the aide and begged her to come at once to take Dad's vitals. Dad wanted to return to the bathroom and somehow Mother and I got him seated.

I dashed outdoors to find help as I was afraid I would not be able to walk him to his bed before he collapsed. Ursula's car was gone. An elderly woman met me next door and suggested that I get John across the way. "He's stronger than I am. I'm sorry I can't help you," she said apologetically. I thanked her and ran across the lawn, thinking it strange that I didn't know these neighbors. From the Guest Room, where I pounded on my typewriter, I could look across to their neat house. Now they were to enter the circle of our lives.

John was tall, strong, capable—and shoeless. "Quick, John. Put your shoes on!" I commanded urgently. "My father needs help. Come quickly!"

I turned abruptly and raced back home to find Mother propping up Dad against the door frame. Wild-eyed and protesting vigorously, he towered over her fragile figure as she tried to keep him from walking back into the bedroom.

"Oh, Doris, where have you been?" she cried helplessly. "I've been calling and calling!"

"Open the door for John," I ordered curtly, seizing my father's arm. Impatient and obstreperous, Dad was getting heavier and heavier. "Let John in! Let John in!" I screamed at my mother. Dad and I struggled together and he collapsed in the hallway just as John arrived in time to ease his fall. We dragged him into the bedroom but couldn't lift him up to the bed.

We pulled him onto a stool and John sat on the bed behind him, Dad's lifeless figure draped over his arms like a rag doll. I rushed to phone for an ambulance. Returning to the bedroom, I tore the bedclothes free, and pulled the heavy mattress to the floor. John clasped Dad around the chest and I held his legs. I recalled a painting I had composed for design class at Boston Museum School, which showed three figures carrying a dead man. I knew now it was my father. He seemed also to be Christ. Suddenly we were all in the painting. Oh, my God! Was this an omen? Did this mean my father was dying?

We laid him down gently and I placed a pillow under his head. Mother watched helplessly. It was all so sudden. It was like a script that was being written, which had to be acted out. I thanked John for his help and he left. I went to the kitchen to make coffee. Suddenly I wondered how Dad was. Mother was with him, but how was he? My God! Was he alive?

I rushed to the bedroom. Mom was hanging up clothes to make the room presentable before the ambulance arrived. I looked down at Dad's immobile form. His head was turned away from me. The mouth was open and still. He did not seem to be breathing. My face registered disbelief, then horror. I felt Mother's gaze.

"Oh, God, no!" I knelt quickly at his side to feel for a pulse. I could find none. I knew then that my father was dead. So fast! Like a knife or a sword of the spirit. First there is breath, then there is none. It was too late.

I lay my head on his chest, crying "Daddy, Daddy. I never told you this before, but I love you!" Was it too late for him to hear that which I had not even known until this moment? I heard Mother gasp. The knife had cut twice. Kneeling above him, she cradled his head in her hands.

"Oh, Bobby, Bobby, I'm so sorry! I'm so sorry! I loved you, too, Bobby dear." Gently she caressed his forehead as she had so many times before.

The ambulance raced up, siren wailing. Reluctantly I left the room to go outside and meet them. Standing in the driveway with open arms I cried out: "I think he's dead. I know he's dead. It's too late."

Two men dressed in white jumped out and hurried in with a stretcher. It's all over now, I thought. I returned to the bedroom. The world had stopped. I, too, felt dead. There were no questions this time from the man in white. Very precisely he closed Dad's eyelids and tossed a sheet over the dormant form. He left and closed the door.

I was alone, in shock, my senses severed. The white sheet was too final. I uncovered my father and held his hand. It was still warm. I pressed my fingers against his forehead, temples, chin and lips, feeling the warmth of life slip away.

"So this is what it's like to die!" I breathed in reverent wonder. "Just the opposite of being born. Now I know the two halves, life and death. Death is no longer a stranger."

"Goodbye, Mr. T," I murmured, studying the high, creviced brow and noticing the fine crinkles at the corner of his eyes, the aristocratic cheekbones, the sensitive hands, long-fingered and artistic, the thick disorder of an overgrown mustache. The intense, almost frightening, brown eyes, now closed, were no longer in pain. The mottled, tawny complexion was studded with tiny brown freckles, weathered by sun, wind and age, as perfect in design as one of our Maine rocks, or the bark of an aging spruce tree. The ears, large and intricate, had been alert to the symphony of nature. Unmusical himself, he played no instrument but created beauty in his house and grounds. After the stroke, music had moved him to tears.

This human frame was the instrument with which he had experienced a life, a vessel with which he had viewed the world. "We are an iceberg," I thought, "seen only in part. The hidden depths are secret and not known to man."

There was a knock at the door. A sheriff's deputy entered to verify his death. The shock of this intrusion sent me into the Florida room, where Mother stood in silent isolation.

"Mother, how did you ever do it?" I asked incredulously.

"Do what?"

"You outlived him! I thought for sure he would kill you first!"

"Hush. Don't say things like that." The ambulance crew was still here. "It was easy," she added softly. "I just prayed every morning that God would let me outlive him so I could take care of him."

Two men placed Dad upon the stretcher and carried him out. He is free now, I felt. Free from his crippled body, free from an angry, complaining daughter and his compassionate, adoring wife, free from the chores and frustrations of everyday living. I touched the foot, the same foot we had so carefully massaged every day for five years, exercising the ankles, the toes, before putting on his socks. Now we wouldn't have to dress him any more. There would be no more of his incessant bleating when he wanted the paper, or a door opened, a curtain shut, his hands washed. No more fights over how to do what or when. We had given of ourselves to the utmost, our conflicts arising, perhaps, because we loved too much.

I thought of the many aides, therapists, doctors and nurses who had cared for him, sharing our heartbreaks as well as our victories.

How many times had I massaged his arm and leg muscles in an effort to reconnect the nerves and revitalize the muscles, trying to motivate his will and stimulate his senses? I reviewed the years of anguish and caring—moments on the porch when he sat contentedly watching the birds, the river, the boats; times when he monitored our putting up the flag; times when we drove him to the beach to watch waves crashing on shore. We thrilled, watching seagulls swooping for bread, or surfers outwitting the waves. I remembered the moments of music, the chuckles over cocktails with friends.

Valiant and persistent, he dragged the dead leg encased in a steel brace slowly around the yard, precisely placing the cane before taking the next step. He was courageous, and he was not a quitter.

"Daddy," I cried silently as they closed the ambulance

door. "I don't want them to take you away from me like this. It isn't fair. All of the years, months, days, hours and minutes ending like this."

I was devastated. I had not expected it to end so quickly. It was too easy. God had surely written the script, for instead of prolonging Dad's illness in a nursing home, he had allowed him to die in the house he had created and loved. His death was like a perfect rose plucked from the vase of life.

It was over. So simple. So final. So complete—and yet so incomplete. Standing on the lawn, frozen and helpless, I watched the ambulance slowly backing out of the driveway, red lights flashing, carrying my father away for the last time.

The warning had been correct, the prophecy fulfilled. Dad had crossed over the canyon—alone.

MORNING AFTER

the sun is shining

        without you

the day is borning

        without you

the clouds are skimming

        without you

morning wakens

        without you

I watch the sun simmer through clouds

    your wife is soaked with sleep . . .

        and alive.

LAMENT

March 1981

So this is bereavement. Deep inside the daily trivia—ashen gestures of getting up, dressing, cooking, eating, reading, talking—lies the unalterable knowledge of death, insidious and all engulfing, leaving you emotionless and immobile. Empty chair... Empty space... The spirit that was there and is no longer.

All of your actions, your words, become meaningless. Part of you is gone, replaced by a gnawing pain each time you see luminous skies that he cannot see. The shock of being here without him is like carrying a dead child in your womb.

Only one question remains: "Where is the one that was?" You are left with incompletions, unfinished moments, unsaid things. The healing takes place gradually around you but inside you are dying moment by moment, corroded by the desire to sleep, to enter into that same stillness—into the forever.

You listen for the wry laugh, the garbled rumble of "Ah's," as he acknowledges your stupidity, your gestures, your desires. You remember the brief smile and the loud protests when something was amiss: the water is boiling, the light is on, the door is open, the sun is in his eyes, a visitor has arrived.

You remember certain smells, sounds, actions: the sharp, acrid smell of a male body; the raucous wail of joy when a school of pelicans flies overhead; the steady dragging of a crippled leg over two acres of lawn. You remember the caustic astuteness of his mind before the stroke. You remember watching fearfully as he reluctantly tries to rise alone from his chair, the paralyzed leg trembling. In vain you grasp for tangible evidence of his having been here. You ache to touch, to hold, to scrub, to dry, to assist, to escort, to exhort.

But your arms are useless. The house is empty. Your mother sits at the dining room table surrounded by letters of condolence, too stunned to realize that she is writing the same people over and over. She needs the safety of letters and loved ones at her fingertips. In unspoken compromise, you avoid eating at the dining room table, settling instead for trays in the Florida room.

It is too soon to assess your accomplishments, to ask yourself if you did a good job. You cannot yet be grateful for the five long years of hiring and firing, running a home. You glance sadly out of your bedroom window. The red flowers he planted spill from the green bush like blood. The orange blooms are tossed about in the wind. A dead palm branch lies on the parched grass waiting to be picked up, like a memory waiting in the back of your mind. You cannot grasp the past and it is too soon to absorb the present or anticipate the future.

You wander from room to room, staring at his empty bed, sitting in his vacant chair. It is like an empty grave. Where has he gone? In your slight hope of rejoining him in a Utopia of tomorrow lies today's strength.

I will live on. I will do my best. I ask for the grace and strength to meet each daily task as I sort through my echoing memories of his life.

RAINBOW

mirage of colors,

gloried down

pure ultra-rays of sun

new found

translucent arc

sky-filled and pure

truculent source of

beauty, sure

the rainbow's edge

    bleeds hearts of care

springing from water's source

    so fair

up from the mist,

    rise like the dawn

eternal truth

    after the storm

THE FAMILY ARRIVES

March 5, 1981

Driving home the day after my brother Bob and his wife arrived, I felt overwhelmed with guilt. Bob had rejected the idea of an autopsy and Dad has been cremated—he wanted his ashes to be spread upon the water. Now I will never know the cause of his death.

Was it a heart attack or a stroke? Was it my fault? Something I did or didn't do? His water pills, did I give him enough water pills? Grief consumed me and I walked into the house crying uncontrollably. "I killed my father! I killed him. He would be alive today if I had given him the water pills. Perhaps if I had never moved him into Mother's room he would never have died."

As my brother consoled me, I thought about the mystery of both birth and death. No wonder there is a God. There has to be, for human kind can't accept the guilt and pain of both creating and destroying life. Someone has to take away the pain, absorb the responsibility, absolve us.

EULOGY

You've gone, a father whom I now hold dear

Your life, once wrapped in embryo of time

My gaze enfolds your quiet face—no tear

Escapes my transfixed eye, now blurred and blind

With sorrow's sudden grief. Deluge deadens pain

And torment sleeps upon my door this night

Remembered for the Light that follows rain

Lost, raging with the elements, my sight

Is dimmed to one small point of Truth—he loved.

Let this be known, Oh God. He loved the trees,

The raging waves, the clouds, the sun above

He loved your world ... and from these thoughts appeased

I now relinquish to that distant shore

His life, his spirit—that mine, too, may soar.

FUNERAL PARLOR

Bob, Mom and I gathered in a small room at the funeral parlor to talk over arrangements and select an urn. Bob, sitting tall and ill at ease, guided us through the conference as though he were steering a sailboat through a rocky pass in Penobscot Bay. Mother scrunched low in her chair, disbelieving and not quite here. I was fearful of facing the funeral service and wanted desperately to be somewhere else. Who would come to the service? What songs would we sing? Could we live through it?

We were asked to fill out a bland questionnaire about

Dad's background, as if he were applying for a job and needed credentials. How formal and ridiculous! Those dull and meaningless facts didn't represent my father. Why must the obituary be so cut and dried, so impersonal? Couldn't I write one with my own flavor ... one that showed Dad's spirit?

I missed Don's presence in the bleak room, a room devoid of any warmth or personality, just like the form we were filling out. Don would have broken the tense brittle spell, adding a touch of humanity and humor, the light touch that this situation so sadly called for. But Don had been unable to get away from his job in Taiwan. Mother, Bob and I were isolated from each other. There was nothing to hold us together. Nothing of Dad, Nothing of life.

We stood up to look at the urns, each one larger and more expensive than the next. "Have you any cardboard boxes," Bob asked. I was horrified.

"Of course. That is the way you will receive the ashes. They will come in two small boxes so you may distribute them wherever you wish," the funeral director said calmly.

Upon leaving, I realized the value of this tortuous formal procedure. The shock of the ritual is needed to force the family to accept the reality of death—and what is to be. A funeral is the putting away of a life.

We were valiant ... Nobody cried.

TO A ROSE

The appalling finality of death

>   lives in the stiff formal arrangement of flowers

>   which greet me in his home.

>   I enter.

Silence ...

>   Silence ...

Silence ...

When will the house live again?

It is not possible

It is not possible

Surely he is in the next room

Surely he will call again

    Surely his loping figure will

stumble

        at the door

            groping for the

latch.

I hate these God-dammed flowers

    only the roses,

        clumped and growing like a bush

            now opening ...

Ah, God,

There is hope. . . again

    what yesterday was a bud --

    now opens minutely

        I can see them glowing

    I can see them growing

        I can smell them, knowing

there is only

Life

Life now ...

Life forever ...

Life after Death ...

sweet pungent

fragrance

Blood-red color of Truth

and

passion

I hold my breath after

tears

knowing

that I must

breathe again

Head bowed at his chair

Yearning to feel a hand caress me --

a little girl crying for her Daddy,

who never touched

her.

CELEBRATION

March 6, 1981

I arrived at the Funeral Home at 3:30 p.m. wearing a bright, green dress to signify new birth. I am full of joy today on this, Dad's "graduation day." I feel I must greet others with his love, for I have reached the other side of the canyon—taking him with me. Fear and anxiety consumed me for these last three days. I have never been responsible for a funeral before and it is terrifying. Will we be able to handle it?

I invited two friends to sing, who had accompanied my religious dance in the past. I was sure that their voices, clear and pure, would touch the hearts of the congregation. I set up two paintings on easels and placed a large bouquet of red carnations and yellow chrysanthemums on a center table at the front of the chapel. Dad's white ceramic cat, the slender one-legged heron, and the tiny, green owl were arranged on a velvet cloth in front of a yellow bouquet.

I bought one red rosebud, partly opened, as a gift to Dad. His death was a single rose, soon to blossom, its essence to be given to the universe just as his children will continue to give to the world their talent and their love. Nothing is lost; it only changes form.

My portrait of Dad looking strong and virile, a brown pipe dangling from his mouth beneath a trim mustache, commands the left side of the chapel. Dressed informally in an open, plaid shirt and blue, V-necked sweater, he gives the air of a stern sea captain. Indifferent to us, the living, he seems to be contemplating new horizons.

My thoughts go back to the time I painted the portrait in a barn in South Brooksville, Maine, while Dad perched on a stool watching my brush fly. I wept when I had finished, dismayed at my ineptitude. After running an errand, I returned and wept again, this time for joy at the remarkable likeness. While the painting obviously hadn't changed, my perception of it had.

At the entrance to the chapel, I placed one of my Beatitude paintings, "For My Sake," showing Jesus standing upon the curve of the world, a beacon for all mankind. Before Him lies a deep pungent blue. In this shadow we can be healed. Christ said, "Walk Thou before me and be Thou perfect." Here, we can "Walk through the valley of the shadow of death," as David sang, "for Thou art with me; thy rod and thy staff they comfort me." I hope this painting will set the mood for a celebration, rather than sorrow. Yet I must allow space for people to experience their grief.

What else could I give to those who loved Dad? I wanted them to be filled—and fed. For I was somehow at last complete. I knew that he did not believe in death; he was too much a part of life. A part of the movement of the grasses, the flight of birds and seagulls, the wind in the sails, the lone loon's cry, the evening sunset's glow; the waning afternoon, the crashing of a wave, the eternal rhythmic flow of day into night. I remembered a poem my grandfather, Henry W. Thurston, composed for his last book, "Education for Youth as Citizens."

"To help develop a world consciousness of kind," he wrote, "I have written two stanzas of a song and chorus to be sung to the music of Beethoven's 'Ode to Joy' in his Ninth Symphony." Perhaps, I thought, we could sing this to the tune of "Love Divine, All Love Excelling."

SONG OF BROTHERHOOD

Men of every race and station

Let us prove our brotherhood;

Men of every clime and nation

Make the world one neighborhood.

Let us tune our hearts and voices

To the tasks for common good

'Till the whole world round rejoices

In the day of brotherhood.

Race and creed must not divide us,

May we feel ourselves as one;

Each with joy of kin beside us,

God a Father to each son.

Let us tune our hearts and voices

To the tasks for common good.

'Till the whole round world rejoices

In the day of brotherhood.

Henry W. Thurston

This song reminded me of my heritage. Although I felt estranged from my father, upon his passing I suddenly knew who I was. For my personality, so unlike my father's, seemed to reflect my grandfather's love for people, for children, and for God. Grandpa Thurston had worked in education, social work, and with the judicial system, lecturing for two decades on child welfare problems at the New York School of Social Work. His books were translated into many languages.

As his granddaughter, I had worked with veterans in hospitals, with children in settlement houses, and with the elderly in nursing homes. My greatest joy had been teaching young people to dance "Twelve Spirituals on the Life of Christ," as sung around the world by Bayard Rustin, a civil rights leader.

I remembered visiting our grandparents every Thanksgiving in Montclair, New Jersey, as a child. Grandpa quoted scripture at every opportunity, reading the Bible aloud, and praying before meals. It was he who inspired me to interpret Jesus' teachings through word, color, song and movement.

The minister arrived a few minutes late.

"Would you like to read my poem aloud, or shall I play the song on my tape recorder?" I whispered hurriedly.

"Oh, you sing it, Doris," he said. "It's *your* song!" I was aghast. The organ music stopped. We entered the chapel and I stood at the back. The minister nodded for me to begin. I flicked off my shoes to ground myself. Crossing my arms at the chest, and bowing my head, I felt my body moving slowly down the aisle as I sang my song, accappella.

TO A YELLOW FLOWER

How did you know, dear yellow flower

When to push the earth apart?

Who told you that the time had come

For you to leave your shell of dark?

How did you know when to break through?

Who told you to push towards the sky?

Will I too, this body's crust, know when

My soul through earth must thrust?

I had written this song for a dear friend of the family, Wells Hively, composer and concert pianist, who had accompanied Lily Pons and Ruth St. Denis. Wells had been my co-worker, when I choreographed religious dance, and we shared many moments of music and beauty.

I had to sing this song for Dad. For all that he loved. For what he stood for and for those who loved him and remembered him as he was. Courage, joy and strength flowed into my body as I thought of all the flowers, bushes and trees Dad had planted and pruned. Even his seed, which he gave to Mom, he helped to prune, trusting that in time and with His will the seed would become a flower, a bush, a tree, providing shelter for another human being.

His was the planting and pruning but the power to grow from birth to death and to be born again came from God. Crossing my arms in prayer I walked slowly down the aisle towards my seat. For five years I had moved as a pawn, at Dad's command. Now I was free. Dad had shown me the way ... Bone of his bone and flesh of his flesh, I was giving him back to the God who made him.

Approaching the altar, I lifted my arms in praise and thanksgiving as my voice rose in victory. It was a conclusion. An affirmation! He was here. He was living in me. Living in each one of us.

Living on...

THE END

EPILOGUE

March 7, 1981

Three days after Dad died, I took an early morning jog along the river in the misty gray dawn. Seeing what I thought was a stick of wood standing upright in the middle of the road, I circled it curiously and discovered a tiny speckled screech owl.

"What are you doing in the middle of the street? You'll be killed by the traffic," I exclaimed, extending my pen. The owl grabbed it with one claw and hung upside down. Normally afraid of birds but intrigued by this helpless creature, I cradled him in my arms and carried him with me. The mottled brown body was still warm and he was breathing.

"He's dying," I thought, "or he would never let me touch him."

I waited for the small creature to turn cold. One green eye was open, staring at me blindly. Feathers stuck to the large, black pupil. The scalloped browns of his body were intricately patterned. Beige fuzz sprouted over the eye rim. The squat beak curved down like a horn.

Suddenly I stopped. My father, the wise one in our family, loved owls. They were his favorite birds. Could this owl be bringing me a message from my father? Was God trying to tell me that Dad was all right, wherever he was? But what about us?

Loneliness overwhelmed me as tears glazed my cheek. How would Mother and I survive without Dad's watchful eye and quick reprimand when we left the light burning, the eggs boiling, the door open, or forgot to take in the chairs?

I drank in the beauty that Dad would never see again. The eerie morning glow of the river reflected the gold and cerise of a coming sunrise. I looked at the placid owl and murmured, "I'll take you home with me and make you well, so you can fly again!"

The owl deliberately closed one eye and opened the other. Stunned, I seemed to hear my father's voice:

"Doris, I will always keep my eye on you, even though I am in another form."

My sorrow turned to joy as I realized my father was with his Father. I recalled the words spoken by another man 2000 years ago:

"Lo, I shall be with you always."

* * *

APPENDIX

STROKE CLUBS

As president of the Treasure Coast Stroke Club after Dad's death, I dedicated myself to building up the attendance through publicity in the press and electronic media. I also invited stroke couples to Dad's home to give them the opportunity to socialize and get to know each other. This group became my team, helping us over the difficult hurdle of the loss of a loved one. Filling up the spaces with love and understanding, they helped me to cross over the canyon of despair and loneliness.

This was my legacy to Dad. The brick discarded by the builders became a cornerstone, so that his illness was not in vain. We held our meetings in various locations—the library, a restaurant, a church. Our speakers included a neurologist, acupressure therapist, chiropractor, social worker, dietitian, pharmacist, travel agent and minister. We had representatives from Home Health, Visiting Nurses and the Council on Aging.

Our club offered the support so badly needed by strokers and spouses. Sponsored by the American Heart Association, the board consisted mostly of stroke patients. As a team we comforted each other, learned from each other and shared our frustrations and problems, our joys and sorrows. New friendships were formed.

Activities included boat trips, theater parties, luncheons, bowling, swim classes and club meetings. Aphasics found comfort in and could communicate with other aphasics. New stroke families learned about equipment helpful in the bath-room, bed-room and kitchen. Strokers compared therapy sessions and followed one another's progress.

In short, a stroke club is a channel back into society, providing education, socialization and recreation for the patient and family. The stroke "victor" no longer feels isolated, as he finds kinship with another stroker, and is able to share the emotional turmoil, pain, anger, helplessness and fear, experienced after paralysis.

The American Heart Association (AHA) and Easter Seals have joined with other health and medical groups in promoting stroke clubs as part of a national attack on strokes.

The American Stroke Association (a division of the American Heart Association), is solely focused on reducing disability and death from stroke through research, education, fund raising and advocacy. The Stroke Association provides information and support, from preventing strokes, to recovery.

The Warning Signs of stroke are:
- feeling weak or numb on one side
- blurring vision, or no vision, usually in one eye
- unable to talk clearly
- dizziness or falling
- severe headache

"Stroke is a 'brain attack,'" a pamphlet explains. "Act quickly and do not wait. Note the time of the incident and call 911 or the emergency medical service in your town. This may be the Fire Department or ambulance. Tell the medical staff the signs of a stroke you saw. You may save a life." To learn more about stroke call the American Stroke Association (ASA) at 1-800-4-stroke. Their magazine, "Stroke Connection" may be ordered on the web at www.strokeassociation.org.

The Heart Association also offers the following guide-lines:

1. Learn the warning signs of stroke.
2. Seek prompt medical attention.
3. Insist on early rehabilitation.
4. Be faithful with daily therapy exercise at home.
5. Help the patient achieve independence.
6. Join a stroke club.

The National Stroke Association may be contacted at 1-800-787-6537. Their magazine is entitled "Stroke Smart."

SPOUSE SUPPORT GROUPS

Attending the first Florida State Stroke Club Convention in 1981, I was thrilled to see over 200 people from stroke clubs all over Florida.

Several very impressive hours were devoted to rapping in a large group of strokers and spouses, led by Dorothy Caspar, a professional counselor from the Biscayne Medical Center Stroke Club in Miami. Emotions, problems and solutions were discussed and experiences shared. The purpose of the sessions was to develop and open up further avenues of communication between stroker and spouse.

We learned that the impact of a stroke in the family produces the same emotional effects in both stroker and spouse. Each is afflicted with loneliness, an identity crisis, fear, anger and guilt. Much of the burden falls upon the spouse who needs support to cope with daily crisis and the emotional trauma of stroke. After the conference, I helped institute a Spouse Support Group for families of new in-patients at Martin Memorial Hospital in Stuart, Florida. The club was directed by a social worker. The Treasure Coast Stroke Club also formed a support group under Dr. Jean Sloan, education director at Martin Memorial. Such groups can be under the guidance of a psychiatrist and social worker or club members themselves. It is important for the spouses to bond and share in their own group, meeting with the strokers afterward.

REFERENCE BOOKS

The following books are personal accounts written by and about the stroke-aphasic victims. They will offer insight and enlightenment to the stroke family and to medical professionals. If you do not find them in your library they may be acquired through an interlibrary loan service within your state.

Personal Accounts:

1.   Armstrong, A.0: *Cry Babel,* New York: Doubleday, 1979.

2.   Beyer, J: *Aphasia: All About Me,* Marquette, MI: Dept. of Communication Disorders: Northern Michigan University, 1979.

3.   Cameron, C.C.: *A Different Drum,* Englewood Cliffs, New Jersey: Prentice Hall, 1973.

4.   Dahlberg, C.C. and Jaffee J.: *Stroke: A Physician's Personal Account,* New York: Norton, 1977.

5.   De Mille, A: *Reprieve: A Memoir,* Doubleday, 1981.

6.   Farrell, B: *Pat and Roald,* New York: Random House, 1969.

7.   Hodgins, E: *Episode,* New York: Atheneum, 1964.

8.   Knox D. R: *Portrait of Aphasia,* Detroit, Michigan: Wayne State University Press, 1981.

9.   Longnecker, Clarence E: *How to Recover from a Stroke and Make a Successful Comeback,* Ashley Books, 1977.

10. McBride, C: *Silent Victory*, Chicago, Illinois: Nelson Hall, 1969.

11. Moss, C S.: *Recovery with Aphasia: The Aftermath of My Stroke*, University of Illinois Press, 1972.

12. Penney, R. V: *Aftermath of a Stroke*, Vantage, 1978.

13. Ritchie, D: *Stroke: A Study of Recovery*, London: Faber and Faber, 1966.

14. Sorrell M: *Out of Silence*, London: Hoddes and Stoughton, 1972.

15. Van Rosen, R: *Comeback. The Story of My Stroke*, Indianapolis: Bobbs Merrill, 1963.

16. Wulf, H. H: *Aphasia, My World Alone*, Detroit, Michigan: Wayne State University, Press, 1973.

Some Recent Books About Aphasia and Caregiving:

1. Adamson, R: *Kate's Journey*, Nosmada Press, 2002

2. Berger. P; Mensh, S: *How to Conquer the World With one Hand...And an Attitude.*

3. Caplan, L; Hutton, C: *Striking Back at Stroke: A Doctor-Patient Journal*, New York: Dana Press, 2003.

4. Douglas, Kirk: *My Stroke of Luck,* Harper Collins, 2002.

5. Hughes, K; Milios, R: *God Isn't Finished with Me Yet*, Nashville, Tenn.: Winston Derek, 1999.

6. Krupnick, S: *Stroke! The Ordeal and the Rainbow,* Gerald, MO: Patrice Press, 1986.

7. McGregor, D: *One Man's Journey: An Autobiography,* Dallas: University of Texas at Dallas, 1999.

8. Meyer, M; Derr, P; Caswell, J: *The Comfort of Home for Stroke: A Guide for Caregivers,* Care Trust Publications, LLC, 2007

9. Mintz, Suzanne Geffen, *Love, Honor and Value: A Family Caregiver Speaks Out About the Choices and Challenges of Caregiving,* Capital Books, Inc., 2002.

10. National Stroke Association: *The Road Ahead: A Stroke Recovery Guide,* Englewood CO, 1995.

11. Parr, S; Duchan, J: Pound, C: *Aphasia Inside Out: Reflections on Communication Disability,* Maidenhead, England: Open University Press, 2003.

12. Parr, S: *Talking About Aphasia: Living with Loss of Language After Stroke,* 1999.

13. Tavistock, H: Levin, A: *A Chance to Live,* Russell, London: Headline, 1991, 1990.

ASSOCIATIONS AND AGENCIES

1.   NATIONAL APHASIA ASSOCIATION
      (An organization devoted to individuals with
      aphasia and their families)
      350 Seventh Avenue, Suite 902
      New York, NY 10001, Toll Free: 1-800-922-4622
      http://naa@aphasia.org

2.   AMERICAN HEART ASSOCIATION
      7272 Greenville Avenue
      Dallas, Texas. 75231- 4596
      Toll Free: 1-800-AHA-USA-1
      www.americanheart.org

3.   AMERICAN STROKE ASSOCIATION
      7272 Greenville Avenue
      Dallas, Texas, 75231
      Toll Free: 1-888-4-stroke, Fax: 214-706-5231
      www.strokeassociation.org
          (Pamphlets; information all aspects of stroke. Pub-
          lishes medical journal, stroke, and "Stroke Connec-
          tion," a magazine for patients and their families.
          National registry of stroke support groups. Holds
          Medical Conferences. Voluntary contributions
          make work possible).

4.   NATIONAL STROKE ASSOCIATION
      (Information on Stroke, Stroke Prevention,
      Stroke Recovery and Stroke care).
      9707 E. Easter Lane
      Centennial, CO. 80112
      Toll Free: 1-800-Strokes
      Web: http://www.stroke.org
      "Stroke Smart" Magazine

5.   EASTER SEALS
      230 W. Monroe St, Suite 1800
      Chicago, IL 60606
      Toll Free: 1-800-221-6827
      www.easterseals.com
          (Easter Seals helps individuals and their families
          with special needs, offering child development

centers, physical rehabilitation and job training for people with disabilities).

6.   NATIONAL FAMILY CAREGIVERS ASSOCIATION
(A family caregiver advocacy, support, and educational organization).
10400 Connecticut Avenue, No. 500
Kensington, MD 20895-3944
Toll Free: 1-800-896-3650
E-mail: info@thefamilycaregiver.org
www.nfcacares.org

7.   AMERICAN MEDICAL ASSOCIATION
(Pamphlets on exercise, losing weight, hypertension, and various aspects of health. Request a list).
515 N. State Street
Chicago, IL 60610
Toll Free: 1-800-621-8335

8.   AMERICAN OCCUPATIONAL THERAPY ASSOCIATION
(A national organization of occupational therapists).
4720 Montgomery Lane
P.O. Box 31220
Bethesda, MD 20824-1220
(301) 652-2682; or 1-800-377-8555
Fax: (301) 652-7711
Web: www.acta.org

9.   NATIONAL REHABILITATION INFORMATION CENTER
(NARIC's information specialists are available to assist you in finding web, print or phone resources you need).
8201 Corporate Drive, Suite 600
Landover MD 20785

Toll Free 1-800-346-2742
www.naric.com

10.   AMERICAN SPEECH-LANGUAGE-HEARING
      ASSOCIATION
      (A national organization of speech language
      pathologists and audiologists).
      10801 Rockville Pike
      Rockville, MD 20852
      Toll Free: 1-800-638-8255
      e-mail: actioncenter@asha.org.
      www.asha.org.

TO ORDER:

STROKE! A DAUGHTER'S STORY: *Trials and Triumphs Caring for a Father with Aphasia,* can be ordered online through the author at *DtStrokeBook@aol.com* (ISBN 1-4120-7875-x), at local bookstores, or from Trafford.com (1-888-232-4444).

Reproductions of Thurston's paintings based on "The Beatitudes" (Matthew V, vs 1-9), are available on *www.artassociatesmartinco.com*, along with her inspirational book of black and white drawings (The Beatitudes: Meditations and Prayers).

ACKNOWLEDGEMENTS

Cover design by Doris Thurston. With grateful thanks to Robert Deckert for his writing classes, inspiration and editorial assistance. Also thanks to Charlene Erlandson, Gloria Kirk, Peggy Meissner, Roberta Synal, Dr. Donald Thurston and to the Writer's Group of South Martin County for their kind assistance. Also thanks to Kevin McLaughlin (founder of Night Heron Poets) and Sheila Rimer, (who published an anthology of "Night Heron Poets") for their continued support and interest, and for voting me "Treasure Coast Living Treasure of 1998."

Special kudos to my poet friends who inspired me: to Anthony Watkins (who published my WAC poems in "The Scene"), and to D. Montgomery, Laura Pyne (deceased), the inimitable Brenda Black White and Art Noble.

And thanks to all the doctors, nurses, aides, therapists, friends and members of Stroke Clubs in Pt. St. Lucie and Stuart (for whom I did publicity), and the struggling Alzheimer's Support Group we breathed life into. These clubs helped Mom and I face our trials, enabling Dad to struggle through his rehabilitation until he reached final "acceptance." They also helped us endure our grief after Dad died, which is when I began this book.

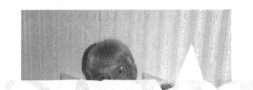

REPLACE WITH COLOUR INSERT

ı
atu
Educ
Mus
Prize.
ter D   ırd
from   as
been ı   ıga-
zine, Saturday Review of Literature, Stroke Connection and
Yoga Journal.

A dramatic series of 20 large paintings on the Beatitudes
has been displayed in numerous exhibitions where they have
drawn critical acclaim. Combining song, dance and art, she
performed from Greenland to South America, moving to Stuart to care for her stroke-aphasic father from 1976 to 1981. She
lives in Martin County, Florida.

ILLUSTRATIONS

REPLACE WITH COLOUR INSERT

POETRY

THE END

INDEX

INDEX

INDEX

INDEX